Peripheral Neuropathy
UNMASKED

Other Books by Dr Brandt R Gibson

The Beginners Guide To Peripheral Neuropathy
Secret Steps To Managing Your Peripheral Neuropathy
Ten Questions Every Peripheral Neuropathy Patient
Should Ask Their Doctor

Fiction Books

James and The Band of Fire
James and The Armor of Solomon

Peripheral Neuropathy
UNMASKED

The 4 Keys To Understand and Manage Your Nerves Better Than Your Doctor Does

Dr Brandt R Gibson

Reach Your Goals, Live Your Dream and Enjoy An
Extraordinary Life Even With Peripheral Neuropathy

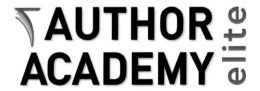

Peripheral Neuropathy UNMASKED ©2021 **Dr Brandt R Gibson**

Published by Author Academy Elite
P.O. Box 43, Powell, OH 43065
authoracademyelite.com

Library of Congress Cataloging: 2021919670

Softcover: 978-1-64746-904-7
Hardcover: 978-1-64746-940-5
E-book: 978-1-64746-905-4
Available in softcover, e-book, and audiobook.

To protect the privacy of those who have shared their stories with the author, some details and names have been changed. Any Internet addresses (websites, blogs, etc.) and telephone numbers printed in this book are offered as a resource. They are not intended in any way to be or imply an endorsement by Author Academy Elite, nor does Author Academy Elite vouch for the content of these sites and numbers for the life of this book.

To my wife that without whom I couldn't accomplish
half of what I do each day.

To my children and grandchildren (current and future)
that inspire me to be my best self in all I do.

To my patients that trust me to help them change their
lives through improved health.

To my God that gives me each daily breath and
continues to bless me with growing insights and
learning.

Peripheral Neuropathy:
Just one more frontier that we will conquer!

CONTENTS

PREFACE

The truth is I could write this as a medical book, even a text-book on Peripheral Neuropathy including thousands of references to articles and medical journals, but that is not my desire or even the need right now. I have been studying peripheral neuropathy since early in my medical education and the depth of study has extended so deep and involved so many studies, books and even personal experience that I have felt overwhelmed in trying to place all this information in a book. I have been "writing" a book on peripheral neuropathy for over 15 years. It is never done because the information continues to grow and change!

I have started this other book and it will be completed at some point in the future, but the documentation process itself has made this task self-limiting at best and almost impossible if I am to do it myself. It is needed and therefore will be on my schedule as I gain the staff and resources necessary to complete the references and resources to make this possible.

But one morning I awoke adamant that a book on peripheral neuropathy must be written as quickly as possible. The information is not being shared and I see patient after patient suffering that have not been given adequate information or sometimes even correct information about their peripheral neuropathy. That has to stop! Therefore, I am writing this book as a resource for increasing your knowledge and information on peripheral neuropathy.

In the process of preparing for this book, I learned that it didn't need to be perfect (it definitely is not) and shouldn't be written from the medical perspective but instead simplified to allow you to understand. I am writing this in the same format that I teach my patients, often there will be accompanying videos that I have posted to improve the information available through the internet when it comes to peripheral neuropathy. Thus, this is not a work for me or my medical colleagues but instead for anyone that has their life influenced or affected by peripheral neuropathy. Whether you personally have peripheral neuropathy or a member of your family does, this book is designed to give you all the tools, all the resources and likewise arm you to fight the battle that is peripheral neuropathy.

That being said, because I am not currently your doctor and am writing everything in a general fashion, there are some disclaimers and legal requirements I must include here:

- This book is not designed to diagnose or treat any disease. In fact, it is recommended that you follow up with your physician before making any major changes in any medications, eating habits or activity levels.

- Although everything included in this book is based on studies published in medical journals, personal research by Dr Gibson and many personal experiences with patients, not all information or recommendations have gone through double blind clinical trials. Therefore, it is all presented as an educated opinion.

- The results discussed in these pages may not be typical and should be understood often as the goal or ideal we are striving for. No expressed or implied guarantees or results have been made or are made by the author or publisher. Individual results may vary. Neither the

author nor the publisher accepts any liability or respon-
sibility to any person with respect to any loss or
damage alleged to have been caused by the information
in this book. Always seek professional medical advice.

With the legal requirements out of the way, I invite you to
join me as we jump into the careful process of *Unmasking The
Secrets of Peripheral Neuropathy*.

A NOTE TO YOU—THE READER

My dear friend, I hope to call you my friend, I have worked on Peripheral Neuropathy for more than 20 years. But the passion started many years before that. Let me explain...

I was very young and I remember lying in a hospital bed. I looked up and saw doctors and nurses across the room with somebody else. I wasn't sure where I was, so I looked around and saw the head of the bed. As I looked, I saw a picture of a skull (knowing what I know now it was an x-ray of my face, but I didn't know that then) and it startled me enough I went back to sleep. I don't remember much more about that hospital visit but I know I went to the hospital twice to correct a birth defect in each eye.

To make a long story short I was cross-eyed at birth. Initially they thought it was a problem with only one eye, but once they fixed one eye the other crossed. Therefore, I went through two separate surgeries while I was very young to be able to see correctly. Amazingly, I have been blessed with eyes that work together, eyes that see quite well and eyes that have allowed me to get through school and become a doctor. Needless to say, this experience has had lifelong influences on my life.

- *INFLUENCE #1:* From a very young age I have always wanted to be a doctor. My desire never changed. My focus never wavered. I was going to be a doctor no matter what else happened in my life! This is what lead me to medical school and

ultimately helped me choose the profession of po-
diatrist. I love what I do and credit great doctors
when I was very young with giving me this desire
and passion.

- ***INFLUENCE #2:*** One of the other reasons I went
  into medicine, and I likewise credit my early life
  experiences for this, is to help people live better
  lives even with health struggles. My vision could
  have been a lifelong obstacle but instead is a lifelong blessing. My hope has always been to give
  people an extraordinary life by helping them manage and overcome any health difficulties or
  problems. This is still one of my greatest desires!

When I entered clinic as a medical student these influences
we constantly on my mind. I loved helping people find solutions and I found great fulfillment in podiatry because we could
often treat or eliminate problems and they would leave without
pain. What a blessing this truly was until I saw my first peripheral neuropathy patient. As I talked with the doctors that
were supervising the students I was dismayed to learn that we
didn't have any good treatments for this major disease process.
In fact, I saw discomfort become a major distraction in patients
lives and ultimately lead to a disability that robbed them of their
future. I considered that option unacceptable and I determined
there most be other options.

With this mission in mind, I have spent the ensuing years
since spending many hours, days and years working with peripheral neuropathy patients, but also researching and studying
options. I have likewise spent nearly $1,000,000 in treatment
options, machines and resources to help find the very solution.

I still spend hours each week ensuring I am not missing something new. I am even more adamant that I find this solution now because it has entered my life personally and the life of my family. Simply put I myself and several of my children have various aspects and presentations of peripheral neuropathy. I will share some of this information in these pages.

So, what am I hoping comes from this book for you?

My goal is to give you the knowledge, tools and resources to take back control of your life. To eliminate the disability, distraction and even discomfort that comes with peripheral neuropathy. You deserve to enjoy your life. In fact, I want you to…

Reach Your Goals, Live Your Dream and Enjoy An Extraordinary Life Even With Peripheral Neuropathy!!

Let's start this journey! Let's give you your life back! I'm ready, are you?

Dr. Brandt R Gibson

PHYSICIAN, AUTHOR, COACH & SPEAKER

Get a Quick Start today with this FREE Masterclass.

Dr Brandt R Gibson is providing you his premier course to help get the background you need to truly enjoy this book.

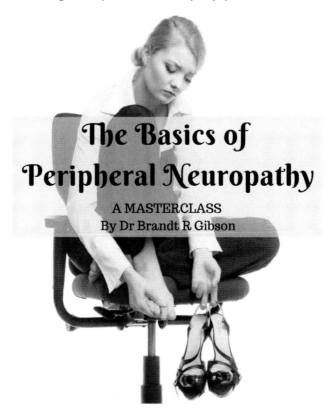

https://www.treatmentforneuropathy.com/neuropathy

INTRODUCTION
DON'T BELIEVE THE LIES ABOUT PERIPHERAL NEUROPATHY

If We Can't Treat It, It Is Only Because We Don't Know Enough Yet!

Peripheral Neuropathy Can Be Treated (But Not Healed Yet)

There is a big misconception about peripheral neuropathy, multiple actually, but the one I am talking about is that nothing can be done, that you just have to live with it. There is really no other disease process that is explained in this way (except maybe terminal cancer). When you get the diagnosis of "Peripheral Neuropathy" you will be either given no treatment options or be offered nerve modifying medications or even pain medications. This brings back memories of being a student in a podiatry clinic and telling a patient about these options:

I was so excited to be finally working in the clinic. I was really seeing patients and loved giving them options to alleviate, treat or often eliminate pain. I saw plantar fasciitis. I saw ingrown toenails. I even so sprains, strains and fractures. All were treatable and most left the office/clinic with significant improvement. But this patient was different. I was talking with my attending and he told me that this patient has neuropathy from diabetes. With the numbness there is often pain and the only thing we can do is treat the pain. The neuropathy was going to get worse and there was nothing that could be done.

As I walked from that room, I felt hopeless. I chose medicine because I could help. I chose podiatry because most things could be treated on the spot, but this was different. How could we know so much about medicine, about health and not have any options for this disease? How could this be true? There must be a treatment for this and I was determined to find it!

Now I could take you through the years of reading books, pouring over journals and articles, attending conferences, working with patients to find options, and even great sums of money spent on treatment modalities and machines to be utilized for my patients. But the key piece of information you need is this: ***Peripheral Neuropathy can be treated!*** That being said, I am still searching for a cure but at least we have options.

Many Doctors Are Wrong

I am going to be very blunt and direct here. First, any doctor that says nothing can be done or nothing works for peripheral neuropathy is wrong! Now I am not saying that they are lying to you or trying to hide something from you. The fact is many don't know what options are available and are therefore missing the information that you need, the information I plan to provide you here in this book. They may be wrong, but that doesn't mean you can't get the correct information.

Second, just as incorrect are all the ads promising healing or complete resolution of peripheral neuropathy. With over 20 years of experience in this field, I am still looking for the magic bullet, the end all, be all of treating neuropathy. It doesn't yet exist and I hope to make that perfectly clear to you throughout this book as well. That being said, with the right information you can find the tools and resources needed to get control of your own disease processes (or even that of your loved ones).

This Takes More Than Medications

Before we even leave the introduction let me make this very clear: *Medications are not the answer!* In fact, although medications can be a valuable interim step for many individuals when trying to get sleep at night or trying to manage the discomfort and distraction that comes from peripheral neuropathy, I often don't recommend we start there. Let me explain a little where I am coming from.

Several years ago my mother was diagnosed with terminal lung cancer. Through the processes of treatment she was given radiation that caused severe injury to the nerves going to the lower extremities (to both legs and feet). The pain was so severe that she would writhe in pain and I knew just what to do. I placed her on a medication, pregabalin, and it helped the pain some. The problem, however, was the drowsiness and the weakness that came from the medication. As we discussed it we determined that the medication was worse than the pain. I helped her work off only to have the symptoms of getting off far worse than the initial pain. As her son I ached for her and was even angry that my "treatment" had actually made things much worse and harder for her.

Now as a scientist I don't make decisions of such a small sample size of one, but she was a good indication of what I am seeing through the literature and throughout the years of treating patients. Medications work well for some individuals (that may be you, and if it is congrats) but many either have poor success, inability to function even with the medications or even side effects that are far worse. I don't recommend medications and we usually will do everything in our power to improve symptom so medications are both not needed and can often be eliminated even if that was a treatment being undertaken before entering my sphere.

Do you need medications for your peripheral neuropathy? My answer would be no! We have better and more effective options for you.

You Are The Secret To Managing Peripheral Neuropathy!

Over the last 20 years that I've been working with peripheral neuropathy, I've seen hundreds, even thousands of patients. And from all these patients, I've learned one big key, one big secret to managing peripheral neuropathy. I'm not the secret to managing your neuropathy (although I can definitely help). In fact, in your particular case, in your peripheral neuropathy, the secret or key is you!

Let me give you a little bit of background here. Peripheral neuropathy is a unique problem, but it is still a medical problem and is similar to any other medical problem. If you are have high blood pressure, there's a medication they can give you. But the key to managing your high blood pressure is you. You must take your medication. You must eat right to not make it worse. You can exercise. Ultimately the only way you can manage your blood pressure is if you are involved.

The same is absolutely true for peripheral neuropathy. Throughout this book you will be given information, resources and even tools, but if you don't utilize them nothing will change. But I want to take it even further than this. Peripheral neuropathy is even more difficult to manage than many other medical problems because each presentation is different, each case is unique to that individual. Your peripheral neuropathy is not like anyone else's! Therefore, you've got to be the one that manage it. You've got to find what the triggers are. You've got to find what things help it, when treatments don't work and when you might need certain treatments. If you aren't involved then our process for peripheral neuropathy management will fail!

Now the last aspect is your personal belief system. If you started this book looking for reasons it will fail for you, I recommend stopping right now and not wasting your time. If, however, you are willing to exercise a little faith, to believe that you can get better if you are just given the right information and tools, this will work for you. I am asking you to step into the dark a little with me and take that leap of faith. I want to give you back your life! Let me introduce you to the system by which we make it happen.

The Gibson Method™

So it has taken me nearly 20 years to pull everything together that we now have. In fact, I have found many options that work for peripheral neuropathy and some options that are not effective or less effective. It is through this process that I created a proprietary treatment modality for all individuals with peripheral neuropathy.

Through this process, **The Gibson Method™**, we have created a stepwise process to diagnose, manage and treat peripheral neuropathy. This is primarily done through four distinct steps.

1. **Understand Peripheral Neuropathy** and more importantly, help each individual understand their

personal neuropathy presentation. So, this is very important. A good foundation is laid by understanding all the intricacies of peripheral neuropathy and then finding the unique features that differentiate your neuropathy from others. Every peripheral neuropathy is completely unique to the individual, like a fingerprint.

2. **Manage The Peripheral Neuropathy Symptoms.** Once you get a good foundation, a good base, and you understand how your peripheral neuropathy is unique, we work on managing the symptoms. Most individuals are seen for neuropathy because of the symptoms that can cause discomfort, distraction and even disability. Our goal is to start utilizing the available tools to reduce symptoms to a manageable level. Many individuals, if treating peripheral neuropathy at all, stay at this step. The problem is that symptoms continue to worsen over time and some treatments that initially worked will stop. Therefore, additional steps are needed!

3. **Control Peripheral Nerve Damage.** Now, I'd love to say you can completely eliminate nerve damage, that's not going to be the case. But there are things you can do to slow down or control peripheral neuropathy in such a way that it is not getting worse and stops progressing. These key steps of understanding the causes of the nerve damage and making the appropriate adjustments can be invaluable in giving you a more long-term treatment protocol.

4. **Thrive With Peripheral Neuropathy.** Now that you're understanding your peripheral neuropathy personally, you're managing the symptoms, and now that you are controlling the nerve damage, we give you the additional daily tools so you thrive with peripheral neuropathy. You get to live that extraordinary life that you were born to live. Although we haven't found a cure, we have found distinct resources and tools that will allow you to live without the discomfort, distraction and disability of peripheral neuropathy.

So the entire goal of **The Gibson Method™** is to help anyone with peripheral neuropathy to reach their goals, live their dream and enjoy and extraordinary life even with peripheral neuropathy! My goal in this book is to give you enough of those tools so you can start on the process.

NERVE HEALTH

PILLAR 1 – UNDERSTAND
PERIPHERAL NEUROPATHY

NERVE HEALTH

1. UNDERSTAND
Peripheral Neuropathy Personally

CHAPTER ONE

WHAT IS PERIPHERAL NEUROPATHY?

Nerves Are A Complex and Intricate Web For Communication, The First Step To Nerve Health Is Understanding The Nerve Itself

There are terms used commonly all over the internet: Peripheral Neuropathy, neuropathy, or diabetic neuropathy, all meaning basically the same thing. The problem is that people often don't really know what these terms mean. They know it means that the nerves are having problems, but don't understand exactly what that term means. In most cases, they think it means the nerves are dead, or they're dying. So what I'd like to do is actually take you through a stepwise process to help you understand exactly what peripheral neuropathy is. Peripheral Neuropathy, by definition is a malfunction of peripheral nerves. Not a nerve death, in most cases, and not absence of nerves except in rare situations.

Before I go into greater depth, it is important that you understand the nervous system itself, including the distinct individual parts so you know HOW the nervous system is affected.

The Central Nervous System

Before you can truly understand the peripheral nervous system, you need to understand the central nervous system. The central nervous system includes the brain and spinal cord. All the nerves of the brain and spinal cord make up this first system. The brain includes all the structures of the brain including the cerebrum, the cerebellum, and the brain stem. As you continue through the central nervous system, you have the spinal cord from which most of the remainder of the body is innervated.

Why is this information important?

First off, none of those particular nerves are part of peripheral nervous system. None of these cause peripheral neuropathy.

Second, many of the formerly recommended treatments for the peripheral nervous system, including such things as medications like gabapentin, pregabalin or amitriptyline which can cause significant symptoms and side effects to the central nervous system. That makes complete sense as the nerves in the brain and spinal cord are similar to the nerves in the peripheral nervous system. Nerve modifying medications will modify the function of nerves throughout the body, including in the brain. Thus we see dizziness, weakness, depression, inability to sleep and other undesirable symptoms that make medication hard or even impossible. Therefore, the central nervous system is a key piece of this puzzle. Treatments need to be understood and evaluated based on how they affect not just the peripheral nervous system, but also the central nervous system.

PERIPHERAL NERVOUS SYSTEM

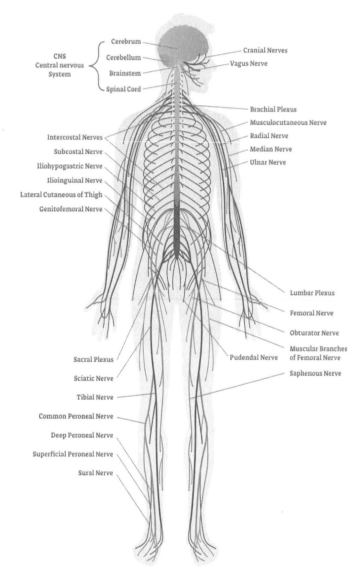

- Cerebrum
- Cerebellum
- Brainstem
- Spinal Cord

CNS
Central nervous
System

- Cranial Nerves
- Vagus Nerve

Brachial Plexus
Musculocutaneous Nerve
Radial Nerve
Median Nerve
Ulnar Nerve

Intercostal Nerves
Subcostal Nerve
Iliohypogastric Nerve
Ilioinguinal Nerve
Lateral Cutaneous of Thigh
Genitofemoral Nerve

Lumbar Plexus
Femoral Nerve
Obturator Nerve
Muscular Branches
of Femoral Nerve
Saphenous Nerve

Sacral Plexus
Sciatic Nerve
Tibial Nerve
Common Peroneal Nerve
Deep Peroneal Nerve
Superficial Peroneal Nerve
Sural Nerve

Pudendal Nerve

Third, the central nervous system is the location of the *Brain Neuromatrix,* discussed later in this book that determines how you both understand and respond to the symptom of peripheral neuropathy. This special map in the brain must be understood to get full control of the peripheral nervous system and all the symptoms.

The Peripheral Nervous System

One of the first steps to understanding peripheral neuropathy is to understand what the peripheral nervous system is. The peripheral nervous system includes all the individual nerves that are not in the brain or spinal cord. So, the nerves of the face, of the chest, the brachial nerves (or nerves of the arms), the intercostal nerves (or nerves between the ribs), and the nerves to the legs and feet. Basically, any nerve that doesn't include the brain or spinal cord is considered part of the Peripheral Nervous system.

Peripheral Nervous System
Somatic Nervous System (Voluntary)
- *Sensory Nerves*
  - *Large Fiber Sensory Nerves*
  - *Small Fiber Sensory Nerves*
- *Motor Nerves*

Autonomic Nervous System (Automatic)
- *Sympathetic Nervous System (Fight or Flight)*
- *Parasympathetic Nervous System (Rest & Digest)*

So the peripheral nervous system is made up of two distinct types of nerves. These include voluntary nerves and automatic or involuntary nerves. The voluntary portion of the nerves is the somatic nervous system. And the involuntary portion of the nervous system is the autonomic nervous system.

Let's start over here in the involuntary or autonomic nervous system. This portion of the peripheral nervous system includes all the automatic or involuntary nerves. The easiest way to divide this system is through "Fight or Flight" and "Rest or Digest." Early in my education process these terms were thrown around to simplify the understanding of the autonomic nervous system. The other names for these two divisions are the sympathetic and parasympathetic nervous system.

The sympathetic nervous system, *Fight or Flight,* is designed to ramp up for an emergency situation. It is designed to prepare to run away, hide or sometimes even freeze. This ramp up process may include an increased heart rate, increased blood pressure, improved focus to your eyes, and even prepare the muscles to be able to run away. It likewise down regulates the parasympathetic nervous system. This is a very important system when functioning correctly. When it malfunctions, as in peripheral neuropathy, it can lead to anxiety, shortness of breath, abnormal heart rate, even the feeling of being jittery.

The parasympathetic nervous system, *Rest and* Digest, is the counter or inverse to the sympathetic nervous system. It will cause decreased heart rate, lower blood pressure and relaxation of muscles. It then causes increase in digestion, improved bladder emptying and improved movement of the intestines. When it malfunctions, it will shut down some of the functions including digestion (your stomach is not going to be have the motility that it needs to have), you're going to have a harder time emptying your bladder, harder time with the intestines (including pain, bloating or failure to absorb nutrients correctly).

Now let's go back to the somatic nervous system or voluntary portion of the peripheral nervous system. The somatic nervous system likewise has two pieces, the sensory nerves and the motor nerves. The sensory nerves are the nerves that provide all sensory feedback to the brain and spinal cord. The motor nerves cause contraction of the voluntary muscles (involuntary muscles are in the autonomic nervous system).

Now let's take the sensory nerves one step further. In the sensory portion of the somatic nervous system there are large nerves and small nerves. The large nerves, Large Fiber Sensory Nerves, are longer extending from the spinal cord to other areas of the body and usually include myelin sheaths or nerve lining allowing more rapid transport of a signal. The smaller nerves, Small Fiber Sensory Nerves, are the nerves out in the periphery, like the hands and feet and are usually not lined with a myelin sheath. Understanding these two distinct sensory nerve fiber types is important to understanding peripheral neuropathy.

Sensory Neuropathy

When it comes to peripheral neuropathy, the most common recognized type is Sensory Neuropathy. In fact, people often go to the doctor because of the symptoms that come from this type of neuropathy. The numbness, tingling, electrical shocks, stabbing pains and even sensations of burning feet or cold feet are all common recognized symptoms. Do you personally have Sensory Neuropathy?

When it comes to Sensory Neuropathy there are two distinct types, Small Fiber Sensory Neuropathy and Large Fiber

Sensory Neuropathy. Bot are unique and both have distinct features that produce the noted sensory symptoms mentioned above. In both cases nerve injury, loss of appropriate neuro-transmitters or failure of the nerve to function correctly can all produce neuropathy. To help you truly understand neuropathy I will discuss both and their associated features.

Small Fiber Sensory Neuropathy includes smaller sensory nerve fibers furthest from the Central Nervous System (brain and spinal cord) and as the name implies are much smaller nerves. Although small nerve fibers may be myelinated, they are usually unmyelinated (don't have the lining or sheath from the Schwann cells) which produces a slower signal than those with a lining. The easiest way to think about it is like an electrical wire that the lining causes the signal to move more quickly down the wire. This is also the case for myelinated nerves.

Okay, back to the small fiber nerves. They carry many different sensation types, but usually are associated with nociceptors (pain sensors). This, therefore, presents with the pains or abnormal sensations called paresthesia (tin-gling, prickling, or even burning). These fibers are the most commonly affected fibers in peripheral neuropathy (especially in individuals over the age of 50). The symp-toms associated with small fiber disease typically includes:

- Burning, stabbing, prickling, jabbing or piercing pain
- Described as "broken glass", "burning sand" or "ice pick to the bone"
- Tight band around foot
- "Pins and needles", tingling or numbness

- Loss of temperature perception

As mentioned above, neuropathy caused by the small nerve fibers can include nerve injury, failure to function appropriately or even nerve cell death (or decrease in the number of small nerves in a given area). This, *Small Fiber Sensory Neuropathy*, is the most common form of diagnosed peripheral neuropathy and will usually occur prior to large fiber disease and often present first in the lower extremities. The usual presentation is in a "Stocking-Glove" fashion or will present like putting on a stocking or a glove (tips of toes progressing up foot and leg or tips of fingers progressing up the hands and arms).

Large Fiber Sensory Neuropathy includes the larger sensory nerve fibers extending from the Central Nervous System. These large fibers are long, myelinated (sheathed) nerves that allow fast conduction of impulses to the brain or spinal cord. They principally carry non-nociceptive (non "painful") stimuli and dysfunction is usually not associated with pain. These symptoms instead consist of numbness, tingling, weakness and loss of reflexes (especially deep tendon reflexes like the knee jerk). The following functions are usually carried by large fibers:

- Motor function
- Balance control
- Vibration perception
- Positional sense (position of a digit or extremity)
- Temperature perception (hot vs. cold)

For neuropathy caused by large fiber nerves is rarely caused by cell death but instead has a high incidence of nerve injury, myelin sheath injury (causing weak or slow signals) or can even be associated with back injury (a common cause of *Large Fiber Sensory Neuropathy*). Except in the case of back injury or traumatic nerve injury, small fiber neuropathy is usually the precursor to large fiber neuropathy.

Motor Neuropathy

The second nerve type in the Somatic Nervous System is the motor nerve. These are typically also large fiber nerves and often myelinated. As such the signals through these nerves are rapid as well. As opposed to the sensory signals flowing from the body to the Central Nervous System, the motor nerves flow from the Central Nervous System to the muscles. Or in other words, the motor nerves flow from the brain or spinal cord to tell the muscles what to do.

Let me explain through a simple analogy. As you start to lift weights you send signals to the muscles causing contraction and relaxation. Through this continuous cycle you are creating greater strength in the muscle that is used. If you stop lifting weights for a period of time the strength will decrease. Muscle use produces greater strength, while decreased muscle use produces loss of strength.

When you get malfunction of a motor nerve, *Motor Neuropathy*, the signal to the muscle is interrupted. The body interprets this as failure to use the muscle and will cause loss of strength (and usually decrease in size). The symptoms associated with this type of malfunction can include weakness, muscle wasting, fasciculations (uncontrolled muscle contractions or spasms) and even some forms of muscle cramps. Although this is often a forgotten piece of the neuropathy puzzle it can present as a major problem and directly interfere with normal function.

Autonomic Neuropathy

Another often *forgotten* part form of peripheral neuropathy involves the Autonomic Nervous System, or the nerves controlling the involuntary or automatic functions of the body. The symptoms of this type of nerve malfunction can produce a wider range of symptoms that are often confusing or are unable to be diagnosed by your regular doctor. The involuntary body functions that can be affected including heart rate, blood pressure, blood flow (blood vessel contracture or expansion), respiration, digestion, bladder function, sexual function and even the simple release of oils or sweat to the skin (sweating happens because of this system). The main goal of this nervous system is to maintain a state of equilibrium or homeostasis where all systems of the body work appropriately together.

A malfunction of this system will either upregulate or downregulate the automatic functions (through the Sympathetic of Parasympathetic Systems) and interfere with the expected or even necessary homeostatic functioning. Although this doesn't happen in all individuals with peripheral neuropathy, it can be very problematic.

Symptoms of Autonomic Neuropathy may include:

- *Dizziness, lightheaded or fainting* – If the blood pressure is poorly managed by the body, changing from sitting to standing or lying to sitting can lead to a sudden drop in blood pressure (orthostatic hypertension).

- *Exercise Intolerance* – If the body is unable to adjust blood flow (blood pressure, heart rate, etc.), for exercise, then exercise will be more difficult or even impossible because your heart rate won't adjust for activity level. This may even produce a loss of muscle strength due to insufficient nutrient flow to the muscles.

- *Sweating Abnormalities* – Abnormal sweating, including over or under sweating, will cause heat intolerance and inability to regulate body temperatures. This can be very debilitating especially in the summer heat.

- *Dryness of Skin* – With poor release of oils to the skin or abnormal sweating, the skin may be drier, may become scalier or even crack.

- *Poor Blood Sugar Regulation* – Due to malfunction of the normal protective shaking mechanism from low blood sugar (hypoglycemia), it is significantly more difficult to monitor and self-regulate blood sugars.

- *Difficulty Digesting Food* – Poor digestive function (including poor movement of foods through the stomach or intestine) can lead to loss of appetite, nausea, vomiting, difficulty swallowing, heartburn, constipation, abdominal bloating or even diarrhea. *This type of Autonomic Neuropathy is often misdiagnosed as other problems.*

- *Urinary Problems* – Due to abnormal function of the urinary tract (loss of smooth muscle contracture), many problems can occur including incontinence (inability to hold it), difficulty urinating, difficulty sensing a full bladder or even difficulty fully emptying the bladder. Many of these problems can also increase the possibility of urinary tract infections (UTI).

- *Vision Abnormalities* – Due to pupil reaction problems, vision is more difficult when moving from light to dark or driving at night. Blurry vision may actually be an Autonomic Neuropathy instead of a need for glasses, especially if it is intermittent and not consistent.
- *Sexual Dysfunction* – Men will experience problems achieving or maintaining an erection (erectile dysfunction) or ejaculation problems. Women will experience problems with vaginal dryness, low libido and difficulty reaching orgasm.

As you can see this form of peripheral neuropathy can be very confusing, can be misdiagnosed as other problems or can even lead to multiple doctor visits without getting any answers. I regularly see patients with neuropathy that don't realize many of the other health problems or symptoms they have are directly related.

The Many Presentations of Peripheral Neuropathy

So, as you can see peripheral neuropathy actually includes a wide range of symptoms and presentations. No longer do we think of neuropathy as only the numbness, tingling or pain that comes from certain types of sensory neuropathy. To truly understand peripheral neuropathy the entire disease process must be understand including the various presentations and the many different causes. There are actually over 150 different causes, everything from compression neuropathy like a carpal tunnel, alcohol induced, medication induced or other forms of toxic type neuropathies, neuropathy is related to systemic diseases including diabetes, autoimmune neuropathies, vitamin deficiency or dependency neuropathies and even neuropathies related to other health problems (think infections, cancer or cancer treatments).

Now that you have the background, let's try to give you a "simple" definition of Peripheral Neuropathy:

Peripheral Neuropathy is a nerve malfunction that can include everything from nerve damage to nerve cell death that is caused by one of over 150 different causes and presents in at least one peripheral nerve area including large fiber sensory, small fiber sensory, motor and/or autonomic nerve fibers.

Although every aspect of that definition can be parsed down to the deepest levels, that is a good basis upon which to build the necessary foundation to go deeper on your personal peripheral neuropathy and associated presentations.

CHAPTER TWO

UNDERSTAND YOUR UNIQUE PERIPHERAL NEUROPATHY

The Truth Is, There Is Nobody Just Like You! Your Fingerprints Are Unique, Your Personality Is Unique, Even Your Strengths And Talents Are Unique. Therefore, It Shouldn't Surprise You That Your Neuropathy Is Likewise Unique To You.

As a young cub scout I was intrigued by the taking of fingerprints one scout meeting. I loved the uniqueness of each individual. Since that time, I have learned we have many other features besides fingerprints that make us unique including iris, retina, the way you walk and personality. Even among identical twins these are unique. Therefore, it was not a surprise to me when I determined over nearly 20 years of working with peripheral neuropathy that every individual has unique presentations and features of their neuropathy.   That is why one treatment will never help all individuals!

Let me take it even further. Because of the unique qualities of your peripheral neuropathy the best individual to find and implement solutions for your neuropathy is you! Through the remainder of this chapter, I will carefully take you through the information you need to determine so you truly can manage and treat your unique peripheral neuropathy better than anyone else can, including your doctor.

Your Perception is Your Perception!

There is a common quote by political consultant Lee Atwater from 1980, "Perception is Reality." Although this statement can and has been argued, perception is a very important concept. Each of us see the world through a lens of perception. This lens gives us our reality that is often very different than other individuals. That perception of the world is created from a conglomeration of our genetics, our experiences, our environment, how we were raised, or religious education and even our individual biases. (Note: I understand that was a major oversimplification and probably excludes some important influences, but the concept is sound.)

Let me attempt to simplify this concept to help us take you to where we are going. In your brain is a GPS, a map that determines how you see the world. This map has some simple features based on your genetic makeup but is otherwise blank. Each rock, each tree, each hill and even each road and building is drawn throughout our lives. The environment in which you live, both physical and psychological, adds to the map. My map growing up in the United States is different than my friends in Brazil. But this goes even deeper. Your home environment, your family, your friends all draw key pieces on your map. What your parents teach you by what they say but more importantly by what they do can change your map. Your belief or unbelief in God or a supreme being will change your map. And then comes your personal experiences, all experiences positive and negative, will influence how your map is laid out. Therefore, as you can see your map is completely unique.

What's on your map?

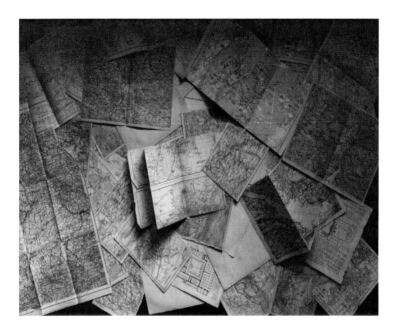

Now that you understand what we mean by "map", I want to take this a step further. There is a concept on how we perceive and react to pain proposed by Ronald Melzack in 1990 called the *Neuromatrix*. Through this concept we are taught that the brains perception of painful stimuli does not result from a simple registration of sensation from a tissue trauma but instead includes an active perception based on this neuromatrix or map in the brain made up of a combination of subjective interpretations of physical, emotional, social and psychological experiences.

Your *neuromatrix* is that map we created earlier. It is through this map, this lens that you interpret your peripheral neuropathy. Even with identical symptoms the perception by another individual with their own neuromatrix would be different. Your peripheral neuropathy is truly YOUR Peripheral Neuropathy.

How Does Your Neuropathy Present?

From your perception, your neuromatrix, we get the presentation that you personally have from peripheral neuropathy. This information is important to help you learn key techniques and tools to manage neuropathy. I will therefore take you through 4 questions to help you determine how your neuropathy presents:

1. ***When Do You Have Symptoms?***

    Most of the automatic or regular body functions have a diurnal or circadian rhythm. This means the functions will occur in a synchronized pattern (day/night cycle). Peripheral neuropathy, especially the neuropathy symptoms will often present in this fashion. Night is often worse, but some individuals also have symptoms throughout the day. Here are the common ways that symptoms present in my patients:

    • Minimal daytime symptoms, significant intermittent symptoms at night.
    • Severe symptoms at night that improve some during the day.

- Significant symptoms throughout the day and night.
- Daytime symptoms but improved when sleeping.

Since everyone is different and every neuropathy presentation is unique, it is imperative that you determine when symptoms are better and when they are worse. You may also find that certain symptoms are present different times in the day (sharp pain at night, aching during the day, numbness when driving, etc.)

2. **What Types Of Symptoms Do You Have?**

As we have discussed previously, there are four distinct types of nerves that can present with symptoms. The symptoms will vary dependent on the type of nerve malfunctioning. Although the presentation is not 100% accurate, you can often determine what nerves are malfunctioning based on the symptoms. Below you will find the common symptoms by nerve type:

Small Fiber Nerve Symptoms:
- Burning, stabbing, prickling, jabbing or piercing pain
- Described as "broken glass", "burning sand" or "ice pick to the bone"
- Tight band around foot
- "Pins and needles", tingling or numbness
- Loss of temperature perception
- *Large Fiber Nerve Symptoms:*
- Balance control
- Vibration perception

- Positional sense (position of a digit or extremity)
- Temperature perception (hot vs. cold)

Motor Nerve Symptoms:

- Muscle weakness
- Cramping
- Fasciculations of muscles
- Muscle failure

Autonomic Nerve Symptoms:

- *Dizziness, lightheaded or fainting* – If the blood pressure is poorly managed by the body, changing from sitting to standing or lying to sitting can lead sudden drop in blood pressure (orthostatic hypertension).
- *Exercise Intolerance* – If the body is unable to adjust blood flow (blood pressure, heart rate, etc.), for exercise, then exercise will be more difficult because your heart rate won't adjust for activity level.
- *Sweating Abnormalities* – Abnormal sweating, including over or under sweating, which can cause difficulty regulating body temperature.
- *Dryness of Skin* – With poor release of oils to the skin or abnormal sweating, the skin may be more dry and crack.
- *Poor Blood Sugar Regulation* – Inability to recognize low blood sugar (hypoglycemia), because the usual warning signs of shaking aren't there.
- *Difficulty Digesting Food* – Poor digestive function can lead to loss of appetite, nausea,

vomiting, difficulty swallowing, heartburn, constipation, abdominal bloating or diarrhea.

- *Urinary Problems* – Due to abnormal function of the urinary tract, many problems can occur including incontinence, difficulty urinating, difficulty sensing a full bladder or fully emptying the bladder. Many of these problems will increase the possibility of urinary tract infections (UTI).
- *Vision Abnormalities* – Due to pupil reaction problems, vision is more difficult when moving from light to dark or driving at night.
- *Sexual Dysfunction* – Men will experience problems achieving or maintaining an erection (erectile dysfunction) or ejaculation problems. Women will experience problems with vaginal dryness, low libido and difficulty reaching orgasm.

3. *Where Do The Symptoms Present?*

The final piece of this symptom puzzle is what areas of the body are affected. Does it only present in your feet? Your hands? What muscles are affected? The point is where do you have symptoms and are the symptoms always consistent in certain areas?

To help you understand the importance of this information let me talk about carpal tunnel syndrome. The presentation of this peripheral neuropathy problem is so localized because it only involves a distinct nerve. When the nerve is released from the compression neuropathy the symptoms improve. Many of the standard treatments for peripheral neuropathy wouldn't work for this entity.

4. *How Do The Symptoms Present?*

As with the other questions, this will vary from patient to patient. The big question is: "Are the symptoms constant, consistent (presenting at the same times or after the same activities), intermittent, or rare. The more information you have, the better options you can find, especially if you can identify key triggers.

One method to help individuals determine "How" symptoms present is a graph that we commonly use in our discussion with patients. Although this graph is not perfect it is very valuable in the discussion of symptoms, especially sensory nerve symptoms.

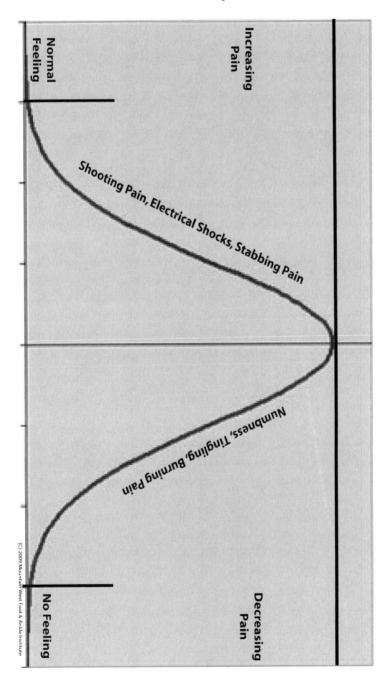

Increasing Pain

Normal Feeling

Shooting Pain, Electrical Shocks, Stabbing Pain

Numbness, Tingling, Burning Pain

No Feeling

Decreasing Pain

(C) 2009 Mountain West Foot & Ankle Institute

As you can see on this graph symptoms can vary from normal feeling (on the left) to no feeling (on the right) with increasing pain as you go up the curve. Most individuals find themselves near the top of the curve and may jump between numbness, tingling or burning and stabbing, shooting or electrical pain. The biggest benefit of this curve is the understanding that often symptoms will increase as part of the process of resolving or improving peripheral neuropathy. Hopefully that graphic gives you a better understanding of your individual symptoms.

What Are Your Causes?

The biggest mistake that most doctors and patients make is ignoring the causes of the neuropathy or even worse assuming it is diabetes (or only diabetes). The truth is there are more then 150 different causes for peripheral neuropathy. Each of these causes should be considered and if possible, eliminated to help you both understand your peripheral neuropathy and ultimately have the necessary information to mange them.

Although I won't list all 150+ distinct causes, I will list the common groups that should be considered:

- Systemic Disease (including Diabetes, Lung, Heart, Liver, Kidney, etc.)
- Infections
- Inflammatory Disease
- Autoimmune Disease
- Cancer
- Toxicity (including medications, alcohol, tobacco use, recreational drugs, heavy metals, etc.)
- Traumatic Injury (including neck or back injury or other direct nerve damage)

- Surgery induced (direct injury or surgery related such as Gastric Bypass)
- Vitamin Deficiency or Dependency
- Allergies (including food allergies)
- Genetic Disorders or Disease

You will notice that I didn't include Idiopathic. That is on purpose. My personal opinion is the diagnosis of Idiopathic Peripheral Neuropathy means we don't yet know the cause, not that there isn't one. My goal is to always find one or more causes to help you move forward on the management. *(Note: Most individuals I have worked with have at least 2-3 different causes, even if diabetes is one of the causes!)*

What Are Your Triggers?

Another big piece of the puzzle for understanding *your* Peripheral Neuropathy is to understand the triggers. I want to include here both positive and negative triggers. What makes your symptoms worse? What makes your symptoms better? This information can be invaluable in learning to manage your symptoms appropriately. Let's go a little deeper.

When looking at triggers, I would consider any products you use (look for nerve symptoms from allergies), clothes you wear (including shoes or socks), foods you eat (sugar, even in the lack of diabetes is often toxic to nerves), activities you do (often neuropathy can be positional). As you look at all these triggers, you can make a conscious determination if any of these triggers should be eliminated completely or if you will build into your routine management steps when these triggers are utilized.

For many years this was a piece of the puzzle I didn't discuss with my patients. I was so worried about treatment options that I didn't give them the tools to eliminate triggers that make symptoms worse. I also failed to look for "triggers" that could be utilized to improve symptoms. I am therefore inviting you to not make this mistake. Log when symptoms are worst and attempt to identify the trigger. You can then start to manipulate symptoms appropriately based on those triggers. *This will give you a powerful tool for your unique symptoms!*

Nobody Is Just Like You!

If this is not yet obvious, I will state it here: Your Peripheral Neuropathy is completely unique to you! There is nobody just like you. Even in families the presentation of their peripheral neuropathy is unique. This is the biggest reason many struggle to manage peripheral neuropathy because no single treatment works for all individuals. In fact, each individual must be evaluated and treated in a unique and personalized fashion. That is the biggest reason you must be involved in the process. *Only you can truly understand the complete presentation and management of YOUR Peripheral Neuropathy!*

CHAPTER THREE

IDENTIFY THE NERVE MALFUNCTION

In Neuropathy The Nerves Still Work, They Just Don't Work Correctly

"If my nerves aren't working, why do I have pain?"

I hear that question constantly! The truth is the nerves usually ARE working, but not as they were designed to do. So, another piece of the puzzle in understanding your peripheral neuropathy is understanding the nerve malfunction. In this chapter I will help you understand more about the nerve and how it can be malfunctioning.

The Nerve Isn't Dead!

I love telling patients that their nerves aren't dead. This is truly an empowering statement because it gives you both hope and promise of treatment options. If the nerves are completely gone or completely dead your options would be far more limited. So, if the nerves aren't dead, why are they malfunctioning? The best way to discuss this is to start with the nerve anatomy.

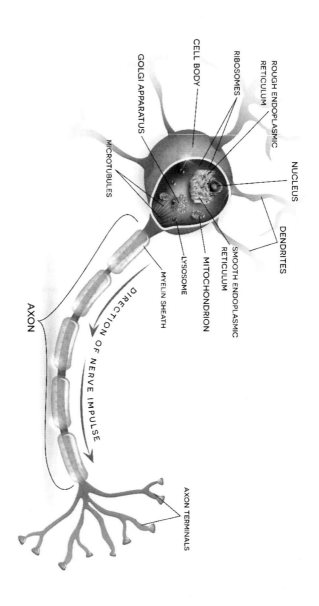

The nerve anatomy is primarily three pieces: 1) The Dendrites – bringing signals into the nerve, 2) The Axon – sending signals from the nerve, 3) The Cell Body – consisting of the nucleus, ribosomes, endoplasmic reticulum, mitochondria, Golgi apparatus, etc. Each is important to properly functioning nerve.

With peripheral neuropathy, although the nerve is not dead, it can be damaged. The dendrites can be injured and not receive signals. Similarly, the axon can be damaged and fail to send a signal out. The axon, however, is also lined by a myelin sheath and will function more poorly when the sheath is missing (weaker or slower signals).

Damage or abnormalities to the cell body can be more significant. DNA or RNA damage in the nucleus, injury to the endoplasmic reticulum, Golgi apparatus or even the ribosomes or lysosomes will cause the nerve to function either incorrectly or poorly. The most common injury to the nerve cell, however, in neuropathy is injury to the mitochondria, the organelle that provides all the "power" or "energy" to the cell. When this is malfunctioning, the cell may fail to function all together or may just be weaker or slower.

As you can see there is a wide range of injuries or damage that may just cause nerve malfunction, but you can also get injury to the cell membrane that may lead to cell death. Small fiber sensory nerves, for example, have been shown to be absent in more severe forms of peripheral neuropathy.

So, when it comes to nerve malfunction there are really only four different types. Any single nerve signal type or even combination of types can present in the various nerves malfunctioning. I will briefly present each nerve malfunction type below:

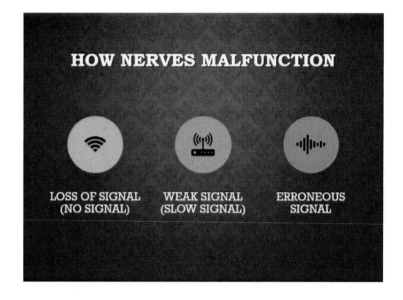

Absent Signal (Loss of Signal)

With certain types of nerve cell injury, the nerve will stop functioning. The most common causes for this include significant injury to the axon (where no signal can be transmitted), injury to the cell membrane or even mitochondrial damage significant enough that the cell doesn't have the necessary signal to function. In some small fiber sensory neuropathies, the nerve itself may be absent. All of these will produce a complete absence of signal or no signal at all.

Weak Signal

A more common presentation in nerve malfunction, however, is a weak signal. When the axon is injured (but not transected), the myelin sheath is missing in larger nerves, the mitochondria is damaged and only providing limited energy, or the cell body is damaged causing less function, the nerve signal will be limited in strength and often perceived as weak by the

Central Nervous System. Because of the weakness of the signal the brain will often interpret the signal as discomfort (pain or numbness) and not improve until the nerve signal strength improves.

Slow Signal

Similar to weak signal, slow signal is also common. The primary reason for a slow signal, that is often seen as weak by the brain, is loss of the myelin sheath, or simple lining to the nerves. The Central Nervous System will often work to "interpret" that signal as an injury or pain because it assumes the slow signal is from a damaged nerve. Therefore, a slow signal can produce either numbness/tingling or pain depending on the brain's perception and interpretation of the signal (the brain map or neuromatrix).

Erroneous Signal

The most common reason for nerve malfunction (or the symptoms associated with peripheral neuropathy) is the nerve sending an errant, wrong or erroneous signal. Although the signal reaches the Central Nervous System (brain and spinal cord) with the correct speed and strength, the signal is misinterpreted because it is sent in a way the brain doesn't recognize. Since the current brain map doesn't have a key to this signal, it assumes again nerve injury and interprets the signal as such.

Remember, that when you are experiencing peripheral neuropathy one of these malfunctions is happening. It is not a dead nerve but a malfunctioning nerve. This is important because a malfunction can be fixed whereas a dead nerve can't be brought back to life (yet). *What type of malfunction are you having?*

NERVE HEALTH

PILLAR 2 – MANAGE PERIPHERAL NEUROPATHY

NERVE HEALTH

2. MANAGE
The Symptoms of Neuropathy

1. UNDERSTAND
Peripheral Neuropathy Personally

CHAPTER FOUR

MANAGE THE PERIPHERAL NERVE SYMPTOMS

With The Right Arrows In Your Quiver, You Can Manage Your Neuropathy Better Than Your Doctor Does

Now that you have a good understanding of peripheral neuropathy and have started the process of understanding your unique presentation of neuropathy, the next step is to manage the symptoms. In fairness, this is the most common reason people present to my office or start searching the internet. The symptoms are ultimately the reason that treatment is necessary. If the symptoms weren't problematic, then peripheral neuropathy would be ignored. In fact, often peripheral neuropathy is ignored initially.

Life is busy! Most of us don't have time for doctors and especially not for doctor visits. We postpone seeing the doctor until the problem starts to interfere with life or scares us enough that treatment is necessary. With peripheral neuropathy the presentation of symptoms usually follows a very simple sequence. It goes from *Discomfort* or symptoms that are uncomfortable sometimes to *Distraction* where the symptoms are enough to interfere with daily life or at least important activities in our lives. As the distraction gets worse, it can become limiting and ultimately becomes a *Disability.* I have so many patients that are no longer doing what they once did because of the disability caused by progressing peripheral neuropathy.

The goal of *Managing the Symptoms of Peripheral Neuropathy* is to give each of you (and me) tools that to get back to life, to living life without even the distraction of peripheral neuropathy. To accomplish this task, we have grouped ALL treatments into five distinct buckets. You should carefully examine each of these buckets and understand when each should be utilized. I love this process because it gives me and each of my patient's treatments at any level or even throughout the day when symptoms change or progress.

I am excited to open this toolbox to you! If utilized correctly it will give you back your life.

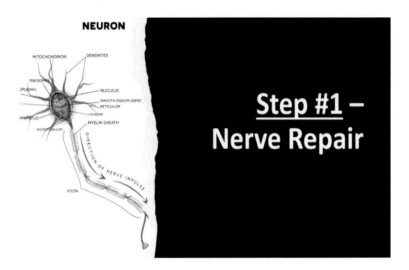

Repair The Nerves

When a nerve is damaged (leading to malfunction), the best management is nerve repair. This is the ideal and the primary goal of all treatments. That being said, repair takes longer and will need to be a continuous, even long-term process. I am constantly looking for new and better options to help you repair your nerves. Just as each neuropathy is unique, the repair processes will be unique to the type of peripheral neuropathy you have and the multiple causes. I could therefore write an entire textbook on the different methods of nerve repair. Instead, I will give you some of the most common and most effective treatments we have found to repair nerves.

1. **Nutrition:** The most effective method for nerve repair is to ensure appropriate nutrition for the nerve cell. This God-given body is designed to self-repair and when the appropriate nutrients are available this repair can happen quickly and efficiently. Nutrition is therefore a key part of nerve repair and includes: eating

right, appropriate supplements (including vitamins and minerals), and appropriate water intake. *A very common form of nutrition is overcoming a vitamin deficiency through supplementation.*

2. **Exercise:** Exercise has been shown to be a very valuable repair mechanism for the body. When it comes to nerve cells, the exercise will stimulate development of new mitochondria in the cells increasing energy level and efficiency of the cell. Improving functioning of other systems of the body through exercise has also been found to be beneficial.

3. **Blood Flow:** Appropriate nutrition is only valuable if the blood flow is sufficient to the nerve cell to carry those nutrients. Poor blood flow is one of the big causes of peripheral neuropathy and doing activities or treatments to improve blood flow can be very beneficial. *Exercise can also be beneficial in improving blood flow.*

4. **Remove Toxins:** If a substance (including medications) is causing nerve injury, the best way to allow the body to repair the nerve is to remove the toxins. This could include just stopping a medication (*only stop medications under the direction of your physician who is managing your disease processes*), removing offending foods, or even a full detox process. Almost everyone can benefit from a detox in managing peripheral neuropathy.

5. **MLS Laser Therapy™:** One of the most effective treatments I have found for repairing the nerves in peripheral neuropathy is the MLS Laser. This is an FDA approved MLS (*Multiwave Locked System*) Therapy

Laser that is a class IV laser and utilizes a proprietary and patented delivery system to synchronize two therapeutic laser wavelengths, 808nm and 905nm. Designed to penetrate the 3-4 cm depending on the tissue type and produce the following biological benefits:

- The 808 nm wavelength provides _anti-inflammatory_ and _anti-edema_ effects via a continuous wave delivery.
- The 905 nm wavelength provides _analgesic effects_, and _improved cellular metabolism_ with potential _acceleration of tissue repair_ or _cell growth_ via a pulsed mode laser energy.

In peripheral neuropathy, the MLS Laser will produce both healing of the nerve cell and improvement of function. _We recommend this treatment as a valuable option for stimulating nerve repair._

As you can see from these four examples, repair of the nerve is usually a process on not just a simple treatment. Repair will often take months to even years to get the desired improvement. Even vitamin supplementation will take 3-6 months to see full improvement. It is for this reason that additional management methods are important in your toolbox.

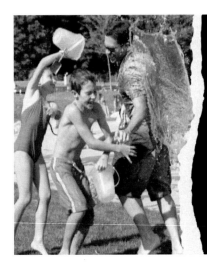

Step #2 –
Nerve
Repression

Repress The Nerves

The most common treatment utilized for peripheral neuropathy is nerve repression. This process consists usually of medications to reduce the symptoms or completely repress the symptoms. The big disadvantage of this form of treatment is the fact that the nerves continue to be damaged and continue to get worse over time. All you are providing is a band aid to reduce the symptoms. Let's talk about some common methods utilized to repress nerve symptoms:

1. **Narcotic Pain Medications:** Pain medications are utilized most commonly when the doctor doesn't know what else to do. These treatments are both ineffective (often leading to 50% improvement of symptoms as best case, but often much less) and problematic because of the side effects. *I don't usually recommend this form of treatment because of the side effects and addiction potential.*

2. **Nerve Modifying Medications:** Many of the common treatments for peripheral neuropathy were created for other reasons like seizure disorder or depression. The goal of these treatments are to reduce the function of the nerves to repress symptoms. The big disadvantage is that all nerves are affected include the nerves of the brain. Common side effects including drowsiness, muscle weakness, feeling out of it and even fogginess of the brain. Care should be utilized when taking any of these medications and also when getting off of them. *Although these are sometimes utilized short term, I don't usually recommend them. You don't have a medication deficiency so let's treat the cause instead of give you another medication!*

3. **CBD:** Hemp treatment has become a new and often more effective treatment for repression of nerve symptoms. There are both less systemic side effects and less interference with nerve function in the brain, making this a valuable option. High quality forms of CBD have little to no THC and therefore are not addictive. *This treatment can be found in both oral and topical options that have both been effective in our patients.*

4. **TENS:** Transcutaneous Electrical Nerve Stimulation has long been a valuable treatment for chronic pain conditions. This treatment is designed to overpower the nerves creating an anesthetic like effect on the nerves. This treatment option doesn't fix the nerve but instead just reduces or represses symptoms. *I highly recommend this an adjunct type*

treatment to help with the breakthrough pain that may cause a disruption in your daily life or activities you want to participate in.

There are a couple unique TENS type units being utilized for peripheral neuropathy:

- *Hako-Med® Therapy:* A specialized "horizontal" therapy that uses a powerful form of electrical stimulation to repress nerve symptoms and stimulate some chemical process designed to "heal nerves." *There are studies showing beneficial effects, but this primarily appears to be a specialized TENS unit.*
- *Sanexas®:* This is a form of electrical stimulation that is much like a traditional TENS unit but penetrates more deeply and is often more effective at reducing pain.
- *Quell®:* This is a valuable TENS unit because it is designed to be wearable and allow normal functioning while getting the repression of symptoms. Although this is still a traditional TENS unit the ability to function while wearing it makes it a valuable option.

5. **Massage:** Massage has been found to be very valuable for improving symptoms. The simple touch causes a release of oxytocin to the body and can increase your ability to function with pain and also can stimulate the nerves to reduce pain. There are

multiple forms of massage that have been found to
be beneficial including:

- *Deep Tissue Massage*: The most common
  form of massage that can sometimes stimulate pain but usually leads to improvement
  of the symptoms of muscle pain or peripheral neuropathy.
- *Fascia Blasting or Fascia Scrapping:*
  These techniques are utilized to reduce a
  perceived or real tight fascia that is creating
  pressure on the nerves. Although studies
  are still lacking, there are benefits shown
  for many individuals.
- *Aromatouch:* This technique is a combination of topical essential oil treatments and
  focused massage. Through the massage and
  the aroma therapy this has been shown to
  be effective at reducing discomfort.
- *Reflexology:* This is a focused massage of
  the feet to reduce symptoms. Although I
  find the science lacking, I have patients
  finding benefits.
- *Bowens Technique:* Use of gentle rolling
  hand moments to stretch the fascia and reduce nerve pain. If performed correctly
  this has been shown to be effective for
  many forms of chronic pain.

6. **Acupuncture:** Although I am not qualified to provide this form of treatment, it can be helpful. Many
   individuals have found great repression (often even
   for long periods) of nerve pain and nerve symptoms

from acupuncture. It is recommended that you find an individual well trained and certified in acupuncture if you want to try this treatment.

7. **Topical Treatments:** Topical treatments can be some of the most user-friendly management techniques for the breakthrough pain. These treatments can be easily carried with you and can be applied quickly. There are really three types of topical treatments:

- *Overstimulation of Nerves:* Many topicals are utilized to overstimulate the nerves and therefore reduce nerve symptoms. The most common would be capsaicin creams made from different forms of hot peppers. By creating a burning sensation, the nerves shutoff.

- *Anesthetic Treatment:* Other topicals utilize an anesthetic like treatment of symptoms. Some common forms include lidocaine creams, Biofreeze™, Deep Blue™ and some other essential oils.

- *Nerve Modifying Treatments:* There are compounding topical medications that utilize combinations of medications that can be rubbed in to both reduce symptoms and interfere with nerve function only locally. This is becoming a more common treatment option.

As you can see there are a wide range of options to manage neuropathy symptoms through nerve repression. The thing to remember, however, is that this should not be the only treatment you utilize because in the long run the peripheral neuropathy will get worse and even these once effective treatments will start to fail. *My recommendation: Utilize this class of management for those breakthrough days.*

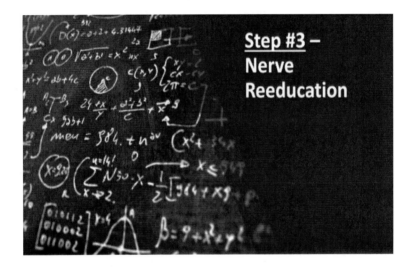

Step #3 –
Nerve
Reeducation

Reeducate The Nerves

One of the most common types of nerve malfunction, as mentioned in Chapter 3, is erroneous signal. In this case the strength and speed of the signal is correct, but the brain is unable to interpret the signal that is received. When this happens there can be significant numbness, tingling and even pain. It is this type of malfunction that requires reeducation of the nerves. This can therefore be a very effective management technique with the appropriate nerve malfunction.

Through the years of looking into and evaluating nerve treatments, I have only found two devices that are effective at reeducating the nerves:

- **Calmare®:** Calmare therapy or scrambler therapy, was the first machine that I found effective at reeducating the nerves. It has been shown in multiple studies to be 85% effective at improving nerve pain from peripheral neuropathy and works very effective in our patients. This is a sequential form of electrical stimulation that helps over a period of 10 treatments to reeducate the nerves and the brain to communicate correctly. The treatment is very effective and shows benefits even after a single treatment (therefore it can be tested to determine if it will work for you). Each treatment gives a longer period of relief (1st treatment usually only helps for 30 minutes to 2 hours, while the 10th treatment usually gives at least 3 months of relief) and return for additional treatments as needed are usually more effective. *I highly recommend this treatment especially for individuals with significant pain.*

- **Rebuilder®:** This is a revolutionary at home treatment! The Rebuilder® has been shown to both *Repress* symptoms and *Reeducate* nerves. This is a specialized TENS type unit with two major differences: 1) It reads the nerve response and adjusts to treat more effectively, 2) The frequency of treatment is in alignment with normal nerve function (instead of overpowering the nerve) and therefore improves function. *Again, I highly recommend this* *treatment for anyone with significant peripheral neuropathy symptoms.*

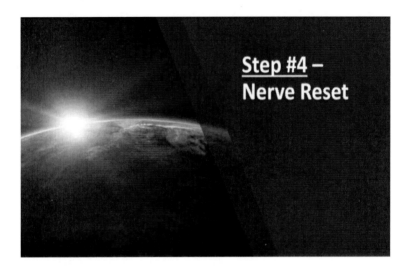

Step #4 –
Nerve Reset

Reset The Nerves

As a software support technician many years ago, we often would start with restarting the computer. It was amazing how many problems could be solved (especially in the early years of Microsoft Windows™) by this simple process. When you consider that the nervous system is equivalent to a very powerful computer, this same process would be beneficial. However, you can't just shut the system off and turn it back on (*wouldn't it be nice if you could?*). It is for this reason that I have searched for a mechanism to depolarize and repolarize the nerves creating the same beneficial effect. I have really only found one machine that truly does this: Neurogenx®. *Although Hako-Med® and Sanexas® may be beneficial, I am getting the best results with Neurogenx®:*

- **Neurogenx®:** This is an advanced electroanalgesic medical device. It is utilized in a revolutionary treatment for peripheral neuropathy called Combination Electroanalgesia Therapy (CET). CET consists of two combined procedures: 1) Careful administration of local anesthetic to involved nerves, and 2) Electronic Signal Treatment by the EAD to specifically treat neuropathy and severe neuromuscular pain. Peripheral Neuropathy improves in over 87% of patients treated. The true mechanism of action appears to be reset of the nerves.

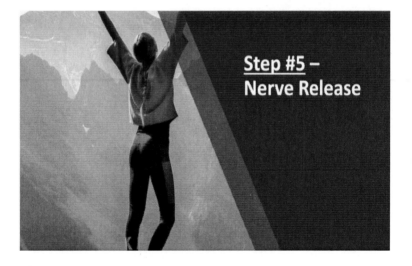

Step #5 –
Nerve Release

Release The Nerves

Although nerve repair is the preferred peripheral neuropathy management technique, nerve release can be the most powerful. Previously we have discussed the powerful brain neuromatrix (*introduced in Chapter 1*), and that gives us the process to *Release* the nerve symptoms through utilizing this symptom perception brain map. Too often we underestimate our ability to control the nerve symptoms through powerful mind-body techniques, but this is a growing science that is producing transformational change in many individuals with chronic pain, including those with peripheral neuropathy!

1. **Meditation:** This powerful technique, thousands of years old, is a distinct process of going into a state of extreme relaxation while focusing the mind on a single idea or even body system. Through this specialized technique, the individual can overcome the discomfort and distraction of peripheral neuropathy utilizing the power of the human mind. The interesting side effects of meditation include improved heart and blood vessel function, decrease in overall stress and deeper oxygen intact. All of these have been found to be beneficial in improving peripheral neuropathy.

   There are multiple different forms of meditation that have been shown to be beneficial in peripheral neuropathy:

   - *Focused Attention:* This is a meditation focused on breathing and the breath. As you focus on breath, all other distractions including neuropathy symptoms can be pushed away.
   - *Body Scan:* This is a type of meditation working to align the body and the mind. This is performed by scanning the entire body for all sensations, discomfort or tension as you scan down the body from head to toe. Utilizing this

scan technique distinct areas of discomfort can be identified and released.

- *Noting:* Another valuable technique that starts focused on breathing or sitting quietly then "noting" each instance of distraction (or discomfort), create a bit of space (move away from the sensation or distraction) and then letting it go. For some individuals this is valuable, but often more difficult to master.

Similarly, there are specialized techniques that can be utilized as part of your meditation practices:

- *Zen Meditation:* This is a method of meditation from ancient Buddhist tradition focusing on how breathing moves in and out of the body. The goal being creating a mind-body connect of "just being". This can often block the discomfort and distraction of peripheral neuropathy.
- *Qigong Meditation:* An ancient Chinese form of meditation focusing on harnessing the energy of the body (called meridians) and sending it inward to produce healing and improved function. Although I don't believe scientifically in the meridian theory of health, focusing energy on a nerve or an area of the body can stimulate healing in those areas. It is this truth that makes this form of meditation valuable in peripheral neuropathy.

2. **Self-Hypnosis:** A powerful, specialized form of meditation is called self-hypnosis. In this nerve release

technique, you utilize either self-talk or visualization. Both are powerful methods of demanding control of the body and especially the nerves. Let me go into a little more depth with each.

- *Self-Talk:* There has long been confirmed benefits of positive self-talk. But this technique is much deeper than just standard self-talk. Instead, you initiate a deep form of meditation where all else is ignored or removed and you focus on the phrase or thought that you want to believe through either *Mantra Meditation* (deep focused meditation with the primary focus being a repeated phrase) or *Directed Meditation* (deep focused meditation with calm directions leading you to the final hypnotic state).

- *Visualization:* This is a truly powerful technique with improvement noted in not just health but also ability levels. The power of true visualization is convincing the subconscious mind that something is real. If done correctly a new reality can be initiated.

For this self-hypnosis technique to be effective the visualization must take center stage with all distractions removed. The movie of the new reality, the new story must be playing in your mind with associated sensations and emotions. The more sensations and emotions associated with the new reality, the greater the reality to the subconscious mind and the more effective the self-hypnosis. *This is the technique I recommend and utilize myself.*

3. **Mind-Body Therapy:** Often we talk about listening to our heart or listening to our head. This phraseology indicates the problem many of us have: "poor alignment of our mind and our heart." Research has made that even more apparent as we learn that alignment of coherence of the mind and body are imperative for optimal function of the body. To truly understand this coherence, you must first understand that the heart, as discussed in the newer field of neurocardiology, has its own unique intrinsic nervous system. Or in other words, the heart functions as a mini brain. Add to this that the heart also sends information and even direction to the brain and the "simple" process of body function is complicated. Only through getting the brain and the "mini brain" working together can the body function at optimal levels.

Coherence: Through specialized training utilizing prolonged positive emotions and simple techniques to consciously control heart rate variability (HRV) and even heart rhythm, an improved alignment of brain, heart and body can be obtained. This new state is called psychophysiologic coherence, or an increased order and harmony in the psychological (mental and emotional) and physiological (bodily) processes. Research has shown the produces both optimal function and greater efficiency in reacting to various stimuli. In peripheral neuropathy this practice can facilitate better function of the brain and body, decreased abnormal symptomatology and ultimately start feeling better and performing better.

One way to help practice or optimize coherence is through working with a physician utilizing the Heart-Math™ technologies. HeartMath™ has been shown to be a powerful, non-pharmological way to manage symptoms while utilizing the heart's intuitive self-regulation to improve overall body health. *This is a good option but can be more costly because of necessary equipment and physician support.*

4. **Be Unhackable:** In 2020 Kary Oberbrunner released a USA Today and Wall Street Journal Best Selling book, <u>Unhackable: Close The Gap Between Dreaming and Doing</u>. Through this book an individual can go from idea to completion at an unprecedented rate. In fact, the principle of *Becoming Unhackable* allows you to use the powerful mind to create "flawless ideas, leverage superhuman focus and achieve optimal performance." As I learned at Kary's feet and underwent multiple in depth trainings by him, I began to see a powerful correlation with *Nerve Release.* Let me go into a little depth here (we don't have the space to rewrite his book here):

   - *Story:* A powerful concept in *Becoming Unhackable* is rewriting the old story into a more consistent new story. With peripheral neuropathy this story could be what your life can and should look like even with neuropathy. By programming this story into the neuromatrix, you can start the subconscious working for you in making this story a reality.

- *Idea:* Another aspect of *Becoming Unhackable* is "flawless idea anatomy." In peripheral neuropathy you create a "flawless idea" that includes the promise of what you life should look like, recognize your success (called promotion in the book) and track your progress. As you track the progress toward your idea (the better life), focusing on the successes not the failures, you will start to accelerate the improvements being made.

- *Focus:* Through specialized techniques of *Becoming Unhackable* you can overcome a distracting world and gain greater focus. This could be focus on the life you want, the life your are experiencing or even just that simple moment. As you learn this amazing focus, you can even overcome the distraction and discomfort or peripheral neuropathy.

5. **Peak Performance (Flow):** Although the science of peak performance or flow is discussed in Kary Oberbrunner's <u>Unhackable</u>, I felt this aspect of *Becoming Unhackable* should be represented independently because of the great strength and value it provides for *nerve release.* In fact, peak performance can become a game changer in functioning with peripheral neuropathy. Let me explain.

   The science of peak performance is based on a simple concept called "Flow." The goal is to access the flow state on demand so that as Steven Kotler says, we can "feel our best and perform our best." Do you understand what that means for the discomfort, distraction and disability of peripheral neuropathy? Through the use of focus, optimal neurologic state and neurochemical access, we can shutoff discomfort or function without the limitations of this discomfort to "feel our best." You can live not just an average, normal or ordinary life but can truly access the extraordinary life even with peripheral neuropathy. *I feel this is the piece of the puzzle that provides the most powerful future options for true mastery of peripheral neuropathy. This is a work in progress but through practice can be a powerful tool in your toolbox!*

Bonus Option:

Exercise: *As a side note, exercise has an additional benefit of nerve release, not just the usual benefit of nerve repair. For example, have you ever run and got what many call "the runner's high?" In this case the release of endorphins can produce an ability to withstand discomfort. Often individuals talk about pain disappearing while they are running.*

NOTE: This is not a primary method of producing nerve release but can be considered as an additional management option.

NERVE HEALTH

PILLAR 3 – CONTROL THE NERVE DAMAGE

NERVE HEALTH

2. MANAGE
The Symptoms of Neuropathy

1. UNDERSTAND
Peripheral Neuropathy Personally

3. CONTROL
Nerve Damage

CHAPTER FIVE

DIAGNOSIS: IDENTIFY THE CAUSE OF NERVE DAMAGE

To Truly Treat A Disease Process You Must First Find The Cause

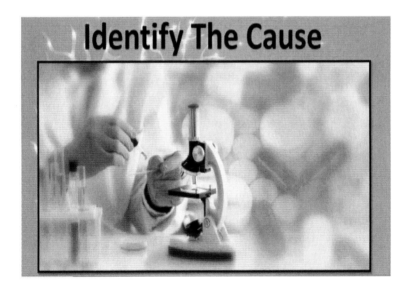

Of all the disease processes in the body, peripheral neuropathy is unique! When you have an infection, they often will determine the bacteria or virus causing the infection and treat it. If you have significant pain from an injury, the diagnostic process is utilized to differentiate a fracture, sprain or strain. Then the appropriate treatment can be instituted. Even cancer is traced to the initial cells that became cancerous because the type of cancer will direct the treatment.

With that all being true, why do we so often treat all peripheral neuropathy like it is either from diabetes or some other unknown cause? Or worse, why do we just assume nothing can be done for it? This is my biggest irritation with current medical practices for peripheral neuropathy!

Let me take this even further. I am going to be direct and may even offend some people, but the truth is that peripheral neuropathy has a cause. There is always a cause! If we don't yet know the cause, we haven't run the correct test. For this reason, I am constantly looking for new and better diagnostic techniques, tests and processes. You deserve not just the diagnosis of peripheral neuropathy, but also a careful identification of the cause (or often causes) of your nerve damage.

Therefore, as opposed to standard practices, we will utilize the same process utilized for all other disease processes when seeking to find a diagnosis.

- First, we *focus on the history* of the disease and any related history that could be aggravating or alleviating symptoms. This is often the most powerful step to help you understand what exams or tests should be performed.
- Next, we should perform a complete or *comprehensive medical exam*. This will provide valuable

information about nerves that aren't working appropriately.

- Third, what additional tests need to be performed? (radiology, lab, muscle or nerve testing)
- Finally, what additional pieces are we missing? It is very important here that out of the box thinking be utilized. Every patient with peripheral neuropathy will be unique. Some diagnostic value will come from this final step.

Let's go into a little more depth with each of these steps to teach you what your doctor doesn't understand, or at least isn't doing to help you overcome the symptoms of peripheral neuropathy.

History

To truly understand any disease process, a careful history should be performed. In the case of peripheral neuropathy everything is important. The goal of this history is to direct the other key pieces of the exam including what physical examination should be performed, what medical tests or nerve tests are going to give more information and what are the probable peripheral neuropathy features expected. Each exam or test should have an expected result based on the history. *The key here: we don't use the exam or tests to get a diagnosis but instead to confirm what the history is already telling us.*

- **History of Present Illness (HPI):** The first step is to get as much information as possible about the "present illness" or peripheral neuropathy. This includes a discussion of the symptoms (numbness, tingling, electrical shocks, sharp pain, shooting pain, muscle weakness, cramping, dizziness, inability to focus eyes in dark, heart palpitations, sweating abnormalities, etc.). It is important to talk about ALL symptoms to help determine the risk of each form of peripheral neuropathy. Then we expand the discussion to when the symptoms are present (intermittent, constant, only in the morning, worse at night, etc.). At this point a basic diagnostic direction is already determined.

As you discuss each symptom with your doctor, you should also discuss when everything started or how long you have had symptoms. Was there a particular event (surgery, medication, activity, etc.) that correlates with the start of symptoms. This is important even if the exact correlation can't be identified. *Example, I had hip surgery and from that time on my symptoms seemed to get worse.*

The next process of questioning is what makes it better or worse. Are there any activities, foods, clothing, situations that make it worse? Are there ways that you are currently treating the symptoms (that make things better)? All alleviating and aggravating factors should be discussed. Through this process you may learn additional information yourself that can change and often improve your daily life.

The more information you can determine (and discuss) about peripheral neuropathy, the more complete the diagnosis and the easier the additional processes.

- **Past Medical History:** The medical history is another powerful tool to understanding peripheral neuropathy. Through this process all past disease processes should be discussed including treatments that have been utilized. Ultimately this past medical history will also direct the medication history below.

  There are a wide range of disease processes that should be discussed here including diabetes (the most common cause of peripheral neuropathy in the United States), so I will indicate the most common areas that should be considered:

  o *Diabetes:* With diabetes being a common cause of peripheral neuropathy, it should be discussed here including all the following disease processed that all often lead to nerve damage and neuropathy symptoms: Diabetes Type I, Diabetes Type II, Gestational Diabetes, Insulin Resistance, Glucose Intolerance, Hypoglycemia and Pre-Diabetes.

  o *Thyroid Disease:* A common cause of peripheral neuropathy that is also easily treated is thyroid disease. With this diagnosis treatment can usually resolve the nerve abnormalities related to the thyroid disease.

  o *Kidney Disease:* The kidney is an important organ for removing toxins from the body. If there are any disease processes in the kidney, peripheral neuropathy can be both caused and aggravated. The common kidney diseases to consider include kidney failure, kidney transplant, Refsum or Fabry disease.

o *Heart Disease:* One of the common causes of peripheral neuropathy is related to blood flow. With heart disease (or circulation abnormalities) the appropriate nutrients may not be reaching the nerves. Any heart disease should be considered for peripheral neuropathy including rhythm abnormalities, Refsum or Fabry disease, CABG, blood pressure abnormalities (high or low), high cholesterol, peripheral vascular disease (PVD).

o *Lung Disease:* Every cell in the human body requires oxygen. Any disease process that reduces oxygen intake will therefore affect the most sensitive cells in the body, the nerve cells. Lung disease process include Emphysema, Chronic Obstructive Pulmonary Disease (COPD), and even sleep apnea.

o *Liver Disease:* Another toxin removing organ of the body is the Liver. Liver disease likewise can lead to nerve damage, especially liver disease, liver cancer or liver transplant.

o *Gastrointestinal Disease:* Nutrient absorption is directly affected by gastrointestinal disease processes. For this reason many of these diseases also lead to nerve damage. The most common causative diseases include Chron's disease, inflammatory bowel disease, chronic constipation, and stomach ulcerations.

- *Connective Tissue Disease:* There are a wide range of connective tissue disorders that have peripheral neuropathy associated. Any connective tissue disorder can cause peripheral neuropathy but the most common include Sjogren's syndrome, vasculitis and systemic sclerosis. Any other diffuse connective tissue disorder can also cause peripheral neuropathy.

- *Inflammatory Disease:* Similar to the other disease processes, there are a wide range of inflammatory diseases causing peripheral neuropathy but the most common include any form of arthritis (rheumatoid, psoriatic, gout or pseudogout being the most common).

- *Genetic Disorders:* Any genetic disorder can be associated with peripheral neuropathy but the following are the most common: Charcot-Marie-Tooth (CMT), Dejerine-Sottas neuropathy (DSN), Congenital hypomyelinating neuropathy (CHN), Hereditary sensory and autonomic neuropathy (HSAN), and the Hereditary motor neuropathy (HMN). There are also multiple genetic syndromes that can be associated with peripheral neuropathy.

○ *Cancer (especially cancer treatments):* Although cancer doesn't usually directly cause peripheral neuropathy, any systemic organ affected by cancer cause lead to neuropathy. The most common association, however, with cancer and neuropathy is the treatments. Almost all treatments for cancer are toxic to cells and nerve cells are the most sensitive. Have you had any radiation, chemotherapy or other cancer treatments?

○ *Autoimmune Diseases:* The autoimmune attack on the nerves is well documented. Any autoimmune disease will have peripheral neuropathy side effects. Some of the disease processes we have found associated with peripheral neuropathy include sarcoidosis, Guillain-Barre syndrome, Sjogren's syndrome, systemic lupus erythematosus (lupus), multifocal motor neuropathy (MNN), chronic inflammatory demyelinating polyneuropathy (CIDP), rheumatoid arthritis and celiac/sprue disease.

○ *Allergies:* Any form of allergy can also cause nerve damage. Documentation of allergies and how the symptoms present are important. Food allergies have been directly related to neuropathy especially gluten (gluten intolerance or sensitivity, and celiac/sprue).

o *Infections:* There are some infections directly correlated with peripheral neuropathy (HIV/AIDS, Leprosy, Lyme disease and Tuberculosis) but there are also multiple toxic effects from many of the common treatments of peripheral neuropathy (even antibiotics).

o *Hormone Abnormalities:* There has been a direct correlation with hormone abnormalities and peripheral neuropathy, especially testosterone and estrogen levels.

o *Other Chronic Disease:* Many other disease processes can influence or even cause peripheral neuropathy including Anemia, Seizure disorder, Anxiety, Depression, Attention Deficit Disorder or Attention Deficit Hyperactive Disorder (ADD or ADHD).

- **Medication History:** Toxic neuropathy is one of the most common forms of peripheral neuropathy (and is often misdiagnosed as idiopathic neuropathy). Although my list here will be incomplete (since it is a growing list), medications that have been shown to cause peripheral neuropathy include:

  o *Diabetic Medications:* Insulin (any form), metformin.

  o *Blood Pressure or Heart Medications:* Amiodarone, Atenolol, Aceon, Altace, Cozaar, Hydralazine, Hydrochlorothiazide

(HCT), Hydrodiuril, Hyzaar, Lisinopril, Micardis, Norvasc, Perindopril, Perhexiline, Prazosin, Prinivil, Ramipril, Zestril

o *High Cholesterol Medications:* Advicor, Altocor, Atorvastatin, Baycol, Caduet, Cerivastatin, Crestor, Fluvastatin, Lescol, Lescol XL, Lipex, Lipitor, Lipobay, Lopid, Lovastatin, Mevacor, Pravachol, Pravastatin, Pravigard Pac, Rosuvastatin, Simvastatin, Vytorin, Zocor (any of the unlisted Statin drugs)

o *Chemotherapy Medications:* Trisenox (arsenic trioxide), Velcade (bortezomib), Taxotere (docetaxel), Eloxatin (oxaliplatin), Taxol (paclitaxel), Campath (alemtuzumab), Hexalen (altretamin), Xeloda (capecitabine), Paraplatin (carboplatin), Platinol (cisplatin), DTIC-Dome (dacarbazine), Ontak (denileukin diftitox), Fludara (fludarabine), Intron (interferon alpha), DaunoXome (liposomal daunorubicin), Vesanoid (tretinoin), Velban (vinblastine), Navelbine (vinorelbine), Oncovin (vincristine), Suramin

o *HIV/AIDS Medications:* d4T or stavudine (Zerit), ddC or zalcitabine (Hivid), ddl or didanosine (Videx EC), ritonavir (Norvir), amprenavir (Agenerase), zidovudine (Retrovir), Emtricitabine (Emtriva), Tenofovir and emtricitabine (Truvada)

o *Other Infection Medications:* Thalidomide, INH (Isoniazide), Cipro (ciprofloxacin),

Flagyl (metronidazole), Levaquin (levofloxacin), Nitrofurantoin (Macrobid), chloramphenicol, chloroquine phosphate, clioquinol, dapsone, ethambutol (Myambutol), griseofulvin (Gris-PEG), linezolid (Zyvox), mefloquine hydrochloride (Lariam), podophyllin resin (Podocon-25), Suramin. *(Note: All fluuroqunilones should be included).*

o *Anxiety Medications:* Ambien (zolpidem), BuSpar (buspirone), Klonopin (clonazepam), Xanax (alprazolam).

o *Depression Medications:* Celexa (citalopram), Cymbalta (Duloxetine), Effexor (Vanlafaxine), Effexor XR, Nortriptyline, Zoloft.

o *Seizure Medications:* Phenyoin (Dilantin), Lyrica (pregabalin), Carbamazepine (Carbatrol, Epitol, Equetro, Tegretol, Tegretol XR), Phenobarbital.

o *ADD/ADHD Medications:* Ritalin (methylphenidate), Adderall (dextroamphetamine/amphetamine)

o *Autoimmune Medications:* Etanercept (Enbrel), Infliximab (Remicade), Leflunomide (Arava)

o *Neuropathy Medications:* Cymbalta (Duloxetine), Nortriptyline, Amitriptyline, Lyrica (pregabalin) o   *Anti-inflammatory Medications:* Humira (adalimumab), cimetidine (Tagamet), Solganal (aurothioglucose), Colchinine,

o   *Other Medications or Substances:* Dapsone, Polygrip, Fixodent, Disulfiram, Arsenic, Gold

NOTE: It is <u>NOT recommended</u> that you stop any of these medications without a careful discussion with your doctor. Some of these medications can have significant side effects and even risk of death if stopped prematurely, incorrectly or without additional treatment options. Please discuss any medication changes with your doctor as I am not in any position to make those recommendations for you!

- **Surgical History:** Surgical history is also valuable in determining a cause of peripheral neuropathy. History of any of the following surgeries should be considered when evaluating the disease process (and possible causes of peripheral neuropathy):
  - o   Thyroid removal
  - o   Kidney or Liver transplant
  - o   Heart surgery (including CABG)
  - o   Cancer surgery
  - o   Back or spine surgery
  - o   Thoracic Outlet Syndrome
  - o   Gastric Bypass
  - o   Carpal Tunnel or Tarsal Tunnel surgery
  - o   Nerve Decompression surgery
  - o   Neuroma surgery

- o   Other foot and ankle or hand surgery
- o   Other nerve surgery

- **Family History:** Any family history is valuable for overall history, but the most important for peripheral neuropathy include:
    - o   Diabetes or pre-diabetes
    - o   Numbness, tingling, weakness, or other nerve symptoms
    - o   Genetic or autoimmune disorders (CMT, DSN, CHN, HSAN, HMN, Guillain-Barre Syndrome, MNN, CIDP, Sjogren's syndrome, systemic lupus erythematosus, etc.)
    - o   Peripheral Neuropathy
- **Social History:** There are distinct social history items that can cause or influence peripheral neuroapthy including:
    - o   High risk sexual activity
    - o   Recreational drug use or IV drug use
    - o   Alcohol use (especially higher amounts)
    - o   Smoking history
- **Treatment History:** The final piece of the medical history is a log of treatments that have been tried, including their efficacy. This information can be very valuable as we move forward in managing and ultimately treating your peripheral neuropathy. It is important that any and all treatments be documented as this gives the more complete picture.

Medical Exam

The physical or medical exam is the next logical step in the diagnostic process for peripheral neuropathy. A full exam should be performed to rule out all other injuries or problems that could explain the symptoms. This exam should also include evaluation of the heart and lungs and the mental and psychological exams. All this information is important in the overall management of peripheral neuropathy.

Additional pieces that are beneficial in peripheral neuropathy include muscle strength, balance evaluations (TUG Test - Timed Up and Go), biomechanical exam (gait analysis, pressure testing and temperature testing) heart rate variability or HRV testing (InnerBalance™ testing or utilizing one of the many health apps found on smartphones), neurologic testing and even tilt table test (*valuable but not necessary*). Nerve testing (discussed later in this chapter) should also be performed as part of this exam.

Power of Lab Testing

A great majority of "treatments" initiated for peripheral neuropathy (including many that can be found on the internet) utilize a process of treatment that I call the *shotgun approach*. Just like a shotgun, where the shot spreads out, many of these treatments are designed to through multiple commonly effective treatments at your disease hoping something will stick. I don't like this method of treatment and propose a more direct approach, what I call the *sniper approach*. A directed approach can only be done through careful evaluation of each patient through lab testing. Therefore, lab testing can be very powerful in management of peripheral neuropathy.

Over the nearly 20 years I have been working with peripheral neuropathy my approach has become more focused and direct. The following lab testing should be performed to help you determine what may be causing the peripheral neuropathy and what treatments are necessary or will be effective:

- o *Vitamin Testing:* Testing for deficiency or dependency – Vitamins B1, B6, Folic Acid, B12, D. *Test Homocysteine and Methylmalonic Acid to evaluate how the body is utilizing B12 and Folic Acid.*
- o *Evaluate Inflammation:* Complete Blood Count (CBC), Sed Rate (ESR) and C-reactive Protein (CRP).
- o *Evaluate Systemic Disease:* Liver function testing, Basic Metabolic Panel (BMP), Thyroid hormones.
- o *Evaluate Hormone Levels:* Especially testosterone and estrogen.
- o *Genetic Testing:* Including evaluation for genetic disease processes and specific genetic abnormalities (including ANA, and Rheumatoid Factor)
- o *Diabetic Testing:* Blood sugar, HgA1c, Insulin sensitivity or Glucose tolerance test (GTT).
- o *Toxic Neuropathy:* Evaluate heavy metal toxicity by blood or urine test.
- o *Allergy Testing:* Evaluate any allergies (especially Gluten, MTHFR)

Nerve Testing

Nerve testing is one of the most important diagnostic tools to determine the extent and types of peripheral neuropathy. One type of nerve testing can be done as part of the medical exam, but the remainder require special testing methods or machines.

- o *Nerve Exam:* Often nerves are not tested completely during the physical exam. In our office there are several distinct tests that help evaluate the nerve function including all the individual nerve fibers that make up the peripheral nerve.
    - o *Temperature Sensation:* Differentiate hot vs cold sensation. *Usually performed with a metal probe (cold) and room temperature item. Many of the original studies were done with test tubes holding hot or cold substances.*
    - o *Protective Sensation:* This is a form of light touch and is performed usually with a Semmes-Weinstein 5.07g monofilament. This produces 10g of pressure to the sites and ensures sufficient sensation to limit skin injury. *This is a valuable test to determine light touch sensation and is usually performed to 10 areas of each foot or hand.*
    - o *Vibratory Sensation:* Vibration is usually the first sensation to be lost. This test can be done with a tuning for or a specialized VPT (Vibration Perception Threshold) device. *This is a valuable test for the initial evaluation of peripheral neuropathy.*
    - o *Two Point Sensation:* This tests the ability to sense one or two points on the skin. This is very sensitive and is often difficult even with very mild peripheral neuropathy. The patient should usually recognize 2-4mm on the lips or 7-8mm on the toes or fingers.

- o *Sharp-Dull Sensation:* Testing of ability to differentiate sharp vs dull sensations. Often this is performed only with sharp to determine pain sensation. *Usually performed to the dorsal foot, just below the ankle, but can be performed to the wrist as well.*

- o *Position Sense:* Inability to feel pressure to the feet or position sense is called proprioception. This can be tested by holding the most distal joint of a digit (toes or fingers) by its sides and moving it slightly up or down. This test should be very sensitive and patient should detect 1 degree of movement of the finger or 2 degrees of motion to the toe.

- o *Reflexes:* Reflexes are valuable as a decrease can indicate motor nerve loss or progression of peripheral neuropathy. This testing can also differentiate upper motor neuron or lower motor neuron abnormalities. *The common tests performed include patellar reflex, Achilles reflex and Babinski sign.*

- o *Additional Tests:* There are also additional tests that are sometimes performed including *Graphesthesia* (ability of the patient to identify characters written on the skin) or *Stereognosis* (ability to identify an object in the hand by touch). *Rarely are these tests utilized in our office because they don't*

> *provide any additional valuable information.*

- ○ *Nerve Conduction Velocity Testing (NCV):* This is an electrodiagnostic test to measure nerve conduction efficacy and speed to determine functioning of larger nerve fibers. The big advantage of this diagnostic test is evaluation of nerve function even at the back (to rule-out back injury etiology of pain).

- ○ *Electromyographic Testing (EMG):* This is an electrodiagnostic test to measure motor nerve function. It is often performed with the NCV.

- ○ *QSART or Sudomotor Testing:* There are multiple tests that are effective at testing autonomic nerve function, including breathing tests, tilt-table tests, gastrointestinal tests, thermoregulatory sweat tests, urinalysis and bladder function tests and others. Many of these tests are dependent on key areas malfunctioning from autonomic neuropathy. Since the small nerve fibers are primarily affected, the more valuable tests (especially in early stages of autonomic neuropathy) are the Sudomotor and QSART tests.

  - ○ *Sudomotor Testing:* Measuring the sudomotor reaction to an electrical current, usually by measuring chlorine ion release instead of sweat release.

  - ○ *Quantitative Sudomotor Axon Reflex Test (QSART):* This is the most common test for autonomic neuropathy and is an effective method of determining sweat gland response to stimulation. This test evaluates the integrity of the sweat release system and measures autonomic control of sweat release.

o *Epidermal Nerve Fiber Density (ENFD):* Through a simple skin plug biopsy, the pathologist can count the <u>small fiber nerves</u> and confirm a diagnosis of Small Fiber Neuropathy. The finding of this biopsy can be: 1) Normal, 2) Normal with degeneration of the nerve, 3) Mildly decrease of small fibers, 4) Moderately decrease of small fibers, 5) Severely decrease of small fibers, 6) Absence of nerves. *The severity of the small fiber peripheral neuropathy increases as the findings progress (from 1 to 6).*

What Are We Missing?

A very important part of the diagnostic process is to ensure that everything is considered. Because there are four distinct types of peripheral neuropathy any and all information is valuable. As a patient, you may assume those symptoms or presentations are unrelated but an amazing number of unexplained symptoms may actually be a systemic presentation of autonomic peripheral neuropathy. Anything that is interfering with your normal life should be considered in the diagnosis of peripheral neuropathy!

CHAPTER SIX

DISRUPT THE NERVE DAMAGE PROCESS

The Best Way To Bail Out A Boat Is To Stop The Leak

The biggest problem with most "treatments" for peripheral neuropathy is that the cause hasn't been determined first. By determining the cause (*as discussed in Chapter 5*) you can look at recommended treatments through what the treatment will do to the cause. If the treatment doesn't *Eliminate, Reverse, Treat* or *Repair* the cause, the treatment will not work for you! That is even true for treatments that have been effective for other individuals. Your *unique* peripheral neuropathy needs to be treated by treating your *unique* cause!

Let me give you an analogy to help in this process. I love to canoe and have taught scouts and youth groups how to canoe. One of the things we commonly discuss is swamping the canoe (flipping it over and filling it with water) and how to empty the water after. One method for removing the water is through bailing (this is slow yes but still is an option). If however you have a leak into the boat (instead of a swamped canoe), bailing will be ineffective if you don't first stop the leak. Likewise, treatments that don't take into account the damage happening to the nerve will ultimately fail and be ineffective (even if initially it appears to be working). Stop the leak (or nerve damage) and then bailing (or treatments) can be successful.

Special Note: Don't confuse "treatments" to disrupt nerve damage with "treatments" to manage nerve symptoms (as discussed in Chapter 4). Although there is definite overlap (especially with Repair) the purposes are distinct and separate and the second will not be discussed in this chapter.

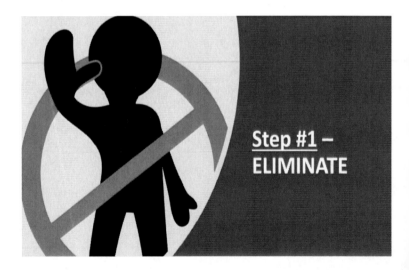

Eliminate

The first step to disrupting nerve damage is to eliminate the cause. Once you determine what is causing the nerve damage, the elimination process can begin. Some common forms of peripheral neuropathy where elimination should be considered are listed below:

- *Toxic Neuropathy:* There are multiple forms of toxic neuropathy including alcohol, chemotherapy medications, foods (allergies) and heavy metals. In all these cases the best way to *Disrupt* this type of nerve damage is to eliminate. Stop the chemotherapy (if possible), stop alcohol use, eliminate foods that cause nerve injury, undergo detox for heavy metals or other toxic substances.

- *Drug Induced Neuropathy:* There are multiple medications (as listed in Chapter 5) that cause peripheral neuropathy. Working with your doctor to change medications or eliminate medications can be beneficial in *Disrupting* the nerve damage. *Remember: Don't stop any medications without working with your doctor!*

- *Compression Neuropathy:* The most common compression neuropathy is Carpal Tunnel. The solution for this type of nerve damage is to *Eliminate* the compression.

- *Other:* Any type of peripheral neuropathy that has a distinct injury mechanism that can be eliminated should be.

Don't underestimate the value of eliminating the cause of the nerve damage. If the cause is eliminated the damage stops!

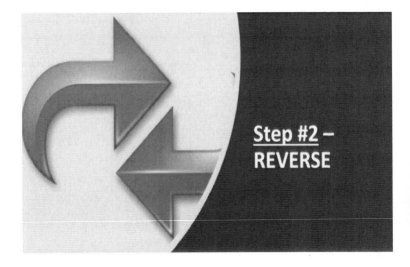

Step #2 –
REVERSE

Reverse

Another valuable step in disrupting nerve damage is to re-verse the cause. Some causes can't be eliminated but through careful treatment can be reversed. The most common are:

- *Vitamin Deficiency:* There are multiple vitamins that have been shown to cause nerve damage when deficient. These include Vitamin B1 (Thiamin), Vitamin B12 (Cyanocobalamin), Vitamin B9 (Fo-lic Acid), and Vitamin D.

- *Vitamin B6:* This is a unique vitamin because defi-ciency or excess can both cause nerve damage. In other words, deficiency must be treated carefully to not cause toxicity.

- *Vitamin Dependency:* A unique condition is en-countered in peripheral neuropathy where through protein abnormalities or enzyme abnormalities a normal level of vitamin in the body is insufficient to provide the appropriate nutrients for the neuron (nerve cell). One example commonly encountered is the need for super therapeutic levels of Vitamin B12 to get sufficient nerve function. Vitamin dependency should be considered with any nutrient utilized by the neuron.

○ *Hormone Abnormalities:* Hormones are an integral part of body function. Many hormones also affect the nerves. The most common hormone abnormality is testosterone or estrogen deficiency that can be reversed through administration of the appropriate hormone.

○ *Nutrition:* Any nutritional abnormality can be *Reversed* through adjusting the nutrition level. This is done through nutrient administration or healthy eating (*discussed in Chapter 7*).

○ *Exercise:* One important activity to *Reverse* nerve damage is exercise. Through appropriate exercise the mitochondrial damage of neurons can be reversed, the negative effects of obesity can be reversed and ultimately neuron health can be improved.

Any abnormality causing neuropathy that can be reversed should be! Don't underestimate the value of this option in stopping continued neuropathy progression.

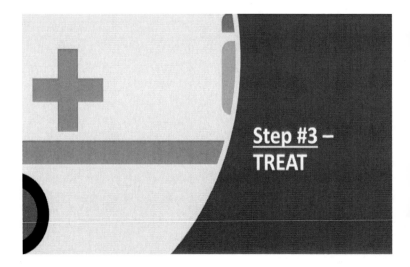

Step #3 –
TREAT

Treat

Many of the disease processes that cause nerve injury can't be eliminated or reversed, so the next step is to treat the cause. The following are good examples of treating the cause:

- o *Diabetes or Pre-Diabetes:* The most valuable option for diabetes (or pre-diabetes) is aggressive management of blood sugars. This can be done through careful eating, medications, exercise, etc. The goal for treatment should be to aggressively manage blood sugar. I usual explain that HgA1c should be below 6 to stop further nerve damage.

- o *Systemic Disease:* The nerve damage or abnormalities caused by systemic disease can be *Disrupted* by treating the disease. Thyroid neuropathy resolves with treatment of the thyroid disease. Similarly, heart disease, kidney disease, and liver disease treatments can stop the nerve damage happening from each of these disease processes.

o *Genetic Disease:* There are multiple genetic disease processes that cause peripheral neuropathy (*as discussed elsewhere in this book*) and treatment of these genetic processes will stop continued nerve damage.

o *Autoimmune Disease:* The autoimmune disease processes can similarly be treated to reduce the damage happening to the nerves. Autoimmune treatments are valuable.

o *Inflammatory Neuropathy:* A common disease process leading to many forms of peripheral neuropathy (including often progression to autoimmune disease) is inflammation. Any inflammatory disease or even inflammation causing disease can be treated and stop continued nerve damage. This treatment can be anti-inflammatory medications, nutrition (especially probiotics), fluids especially water and rest/sleep. *Since inflammation leads to so many other disease processes this is a valuable option to reduce peripheral neuropathy symptoms and stop further nerve damage,*

o *Vascular Disease:* Blood flow is imperative for cell health, especially for a very sensitive neuron. If there is vascular disease including atherosclerosis, cholesterol problems, anemia, peripheral vascular disease (PVD), venous stasis disease or even edema, there will likewise be continued nerve injury. By treating these disease processes (and repairing when necessary), nerve injury progression can be stopped.

o *Back Injury:* Nerve compression or pain associated with spinal or back abnormalities can usually be treated. These treatments can include surgical treatments, but my recommendations are actually through specialized exercises and treatments studied and perfected by Dr Stuart McGill. I have taken the time to become educated in his methods and techniques. Through his treatments back pain (and the associated nerve damage) can be alleviated, and continued nerve damage can be stopped. (*Additional information on his system can be found in his books <u>Back Mechanics</u> and <u>Ultimate Back Fitness and Performance</u>.*)

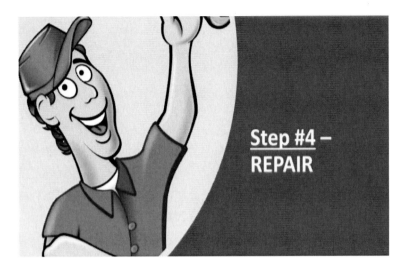

Repair

Although repair is typically instituted in many of the neuropathy types, there are certain causes of peripheral neuropathy that repair is the only option. Nerve repair can be done in situations involving trauma, blood flow abnormalities, different types of nerve injury and even loss of myelin sheath or neurotransmitters. In all cases repair can both allow the nerve to function more appropriately and stop additional nerve damage. (*See Chapter 4 for common nerve repair methods.*)

Finding The Best Treatments

The good news about these four treatment steps to *Disrupt* the nerve damage is that all effective treatments will fit into one of these buckets. If the treatment doesn't eliminate, reverse, treat or repair the nerves, the treatment will be ineffective and is a waste of money. As I look at new treatments, I am making the same assessment. If it doesn't do one of these four things it will not provide long-term benefits for peripheral neuropathy.

So to find the best treatments, you should *Diagnose* the cause and then utilize Eliminate, Reverse, Treat or Repair to *Disrupt* (or stop) that cause. Through this simple process you can quickly pick the appropriate treatment for your peripheral neuropathy.

CHAPTER SEVEN

DETER CONTINUED NERVE DAMAGE

Healthy Habits Lead To Healthy Nerves

The final step to *Control Nerve Damage* is to put into place a regimen that is designed to *Deter* (or prevent) further nerve damage. By improving daily habits, the nerve health can be improved significantly, and the body can be optimized to assist in nerve repair, nerve treatment and even neuroprotection (nerve protection). Our goal is to help you prevent further nerve injury or nerve damage by utilizing 5 healthy habits in your daily life. Each habit is beneficial to the nerves, but as a conglomerate they are truly transformational.

Healthy Eating

I often joke that eating is one of my talents and I practice it every day to ensure God doesn't take it away. The truth is many of us spend time throughout every day eating. Whether truly a talent, a habit or just a necessity, the way that we eat can have a powerful influence on our overall health. For this reason,

I have spent much of my adult life trying to find the best ways to optimize how I eat without limiting those special moments or those family times where eating can be enjoyable. I don't want to take away that enjoyment from myself or any of my patients. My goal is to find an eating "lifestyle" that allows leeway while still providing the necessary tools for health. It is for this reason that I have researched and attempted an amazing number of eating programs or diets.

I have implemented calorie limitations, intermittent fasting, Atkins diet, Carbohydrate addict diets (low-carb diets), keto, paleo, plant-based diets, low-fat diets, the Mediterranean diet and many modifications of each. I have eliminated sugar and increased exercise. All provided varying degrees of health and even weight loss, but my best indication of efficacy of each was how I felt. My opinion is that any "eating program" should give me the ability to go out to eat, to enjoy family and even treats if desired, allow me the energy I desire and ultimately help me maintain my activity level while also producing a healthy weight. It was this goal that caused me to start to create an eating program that when tested was very effective. I will introduce that first, and then I will explain what I am utilizing now for my patients (especially those with peripheral neuropathy).

- *Nature's 8™* – The key nutrients needed by every individual come through two distinct food groups primarily (vegetables and fruits). Therefore, I based this new eating program on these food groups. *As part of Nature's 8™ there are 8 distinct pieces:*
    1. **The Cleanse:** Initiate with a Cleanse to kick start the health. Every program that I

have seen with success requires a period of cleanse.

- Over the period of 3 Days.
- Eliminate all fluids except water (No juices, No soft drinks, No Milk), but you should drink 10-12 cups of water a day.
- Eliminate all sugar containing foods. *You can be as strict as you like, but deserts are definitely out. Natural sugars (as in fruits) are okay.*
- Intermittent Fasting : Recommend eating in a 6 hour period each day (18 hours of fasting, then 6 hours of eating). *If you want to be more extreme, you can start with a 24 – 48 hour fast.* Focus on continuing to drink fluids throughout the fast.
- No processed foods. No diary. No breads or cereals. Eating should focus on vegetables with some fruits.

2. **Fluids:** It is imperative that fluids become an active part of your nutrition plan. Drink 8-10 cups of water per day. That is in addition to any other fluids that you drink.

3. **Vegetables:** Vegetables should be the primary portion of your meals, with a focus on getting 6-8 servings of vegetables per day. Counting is not important, but focusing on vegetables will guarantee a much higher

level of health and improved functioning of all systems in the body especially nerves.

4. **Fruits:** Fruits are usually the easiest nutrient rich food to eat and should be a key part of any meal plan. Eat <u>6-8 servings of fruit per day</u>. Focus on berries where possible, but an apple a day is also valuable.

5. **Period of Fasting:** Intermittent fasting has been shown to be beneficial to many individuals seeking to improve health. This is not a lifestyle many individuals can do. My recommendation is no eating (Fasting) between 7:00pm and 7:00am. This period of recovery and renewal is an important part of metabolism, blood sugar maintenance and provides energy during periods of activity. *Special occasions can allow eating outside this period, but after 7:00pm should not be the norm.*

6. **Limit Sugars:** Sugar containing foods (treats, desserts, etc.) have been shown to be damaging to nerve cells and in some cases can be poisonous. By limiting sugars (not including natural sugars like fruits or honey) you will see a quick improvement in health and ultimately some improvement in Peripheral Neuropathy.

7. **Limit Processed Foods:** One of the biggest detrimental effects of today's diet is processed foods. The more processed the food, the less nutrition is obtained from the

food. Many of the negative health presentations today can be traced to eating highly
processed foods.

8. **Limit Snacks:** Snacks are usually foods we
   wouldn't normally eat. There is also a
   medical benefit to not eating between
   meals. The science states that blood sugars
   normalize and metabolism is better if you
   aren't eating between your usual 3 meals
   (Breakfast, Lunch & Dinner)

This works and has been very valuable to many of
my patients in improving health. It is not, however,
the most effective eating program that I have found.

- *The 7 Systems Plan™* - Dr Pat Luse over a period
  or over 30 years has created a program that is designed to optimize the science of health to improve
  the function of the "7 Systems" of the body. His
  award-winning book, *7 Systems Plan* and the associated course continues to transform lives and
  produce amazing health.

  I have personally worked with him in imple-
  menting this program for my patients and am now
  using it myself to create the long-term health I am
  also seeking. Although I won't attempt to reproduce
  his content here, I do recommend both his book and
  I would be happy to coach you through his program
  (see links at the end of this book). Here are some
  key highlights:

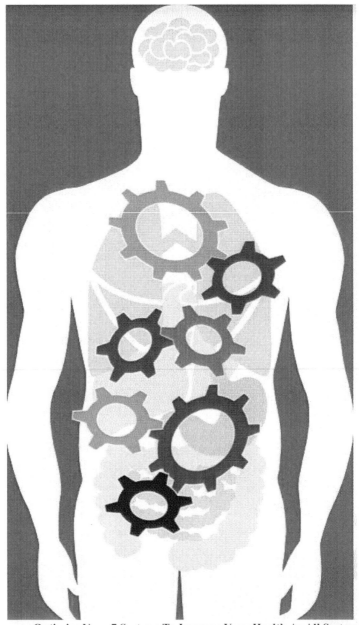

**Optimize Your 7 Systems To Improve Your Health As All Systems
Start To Work In Perfect Unison**
Used by permission from *7 Systems Plan* by Dr Pat Luse

1. *The Structural System* – Fat, Muscle and Bone optimization to build strong bones, gain muscle and reduce excess fat. *Through proper structure, many symptoms of peripheral neuropathy can be reduced.*

2. *The Digestive System* – Optimize digestion including being satisfied with less food, proper gut bacteria health, and optimizing gut function including proper gut and brain communication. *The key to proper nutrition for the nerves is proper digestive system function.*

3. *The Delivery System* – Optimizing the delivery of nutrients throughout the body (including heart, blood flow and lymphatic flow). *For nerve health the nutrients must be carried to the neuron (nerve cell) efficiently.*

4. *The Energy System* – Increase energy while optimizing cell health (very valuable for nerve health) and proper exercise modalities and techniques. *This system is invaluable for improving neuron function and optimizing exercise.*

5. *The Communication System* – Improve communication in the body through nerves and neurotransmitters and hormones. *This*

also focuses on stress reduction as a powerful health technique.

6. The Defense System – A key piece of overall body health is the defense system. By optimizing this system, you can reduce allergies, asthma, inflammation and auto-immune symptoms. *Nerve repair and prevention of further nerve damage requires optimal health of this system.*

7. The Detox System – Toxic damage is happening throughout the body. Optimizing this system will improve all systems of the body and allow proper healing. *For peripheral neuropathy this is an invaluable process to remove many of the damaging substances from the body.*

Finding the program that helps you optimize your health will be one of the most valuable methods for preventing further nerve damage and ultimately improve nerve health.

Don't Forget The Water

In the human body approximately 60% is made up of water. In fact, H.H. Mitchell noted in Journal of Biological Chemistry 158, found that the brain consists of 73% water. This indicates the great value water has in the function of the nervous system. When you go down to the cellular level, many of the functions of the cell require water. For the neuron (the nerve cell) to function properly sufficient water must be available.

With that understanding one of the key puzzle pieces in deterring or preventing nerve damage is fluid intake. Not just any fluid, however, but water to be exact. Most individuals will recommend 8 cups of water a day. With peripheral neuropathy I am now suggesting 12 cups of water a day to ensure sufficient for cellular function, proper digestion, sufficient ability to detox the tissues, rich blood flow and hydration levels that produce greater health. *Please make this a consistent and regular part of your daily routine!*

Regular Exercise

The value of exercise is not in question. In fact, many studies have been done over many years directly correlating health with exercise. That being said, peripheral neuropathy makes exercise more difficult and often can produce discomfort or even disability limiting the ability to exercise. Regular exercise, however, is imperative to prevent further nerve damage.

The type of exercise is not important but the improvement of blood flow, increased heart health and even cellular health from improved energy levels is a key. Mitochondria, the power plant for the cells, are tripled as least through the simple act of exercise. Any exercise can be valuable, even simple walking (get in your steps). My recommendation is to find something you can do and create a step goal or a 20-30 minute period at least 5-6 times a week where you do regular exercise. There are so many options that can be done even with peripheral neuropathy. *If you really want to deter or prevent nerve damage, find a way to exercise regularly.*

The Power of Sleep

If you talk to my children, they will agree that I often joke "Sleep is overrated!" The truth is, however, the value of sleep is not in question. Studies now show that sleep is directly related to nerve pain and peripheral neuropathy symptoms. Sleep is also related to overall health and wellness. To deter or prevent nerve damage then appropriate sleep should be a regular part of your life.

In all the studies I have reviewed, optimal sleep is between 7-8 hours, less or more can both be problematic. Some individuals may require less sleep but for most individuals this amount of sleep is necessary for reset of the body systems and to optimize healthy healing of all areas of the body. *Don't underestimate the value of body "reset" through proper sleep.*

Daily Lifestyle

I tell my 11 children on a regular basis that nobody can make you mad, make your sad or hurt your feelings. This only happens if you give them the power over your life. The final step to *Deter* nerve damage is to create a positive daily lifestyle. I am not just talking about living as if everything is easy or as if peripheral neuropathy doesn't cause discomfort, distraction and even some disability. In fact, I recognize that often you haven't been able to live the life you want to live. That is why we are actively treating peripheral neuropathy. What I am saying is that you need to take control of your daily lifestyle!

Let me explain a little more. Through a portion of your brain called the RAS filter, the reticular activating system, your brain is constantly filtering out "the noise". The conscious mind will only see what is considered important. The RAS filter is tasked by the subconscious mind to only show the conscious mind what it determines is important. Similar to the social media platforms and the internet search engines showing you what you showed previous interest in, the RAS filter will do the same. This is why you will "see" what you are looking for. If you look for the bad, you find the bad. If you look for the good, you will find the good. *This is truly a powerful concept!*

My invitation, therefore, is to look for the blessings, the ways your nerves are functioning better, the periods of time or activities that weren't interrupted by nerve symptoms and ultimately you will start to notice more of this. Studies have even shown individuals that focus on the positive aspects of life have improved overall health. Your mind is truly powerful and can heal much more effectively than any medicine or medical treatment.

Deter or prevent additional nerve damage by focusing on the progress you are making, the activities you have returned to, the symptoms that have disappeared. You will be amazed!

NERVE HEALTH

PILLAR 4 – THRIVE WITH PERIPHERAL NEUROPATHY

NERVE HEALTH

1. UNDERSTAND
Peripheral Neuropathy Personally

2. MANAGE
The Symptoms of Neuropathy

3. CONTROL
Nerve Damage

4. THRIVE
With Peripheral Neuropathy

CHAPTER EIGHT

4 SECRETS TO THRIVE WITH PERIPHERAL NEUROPATHY

As You Align Each Intricate Aspect Of Health In Your Life, You Will Find Greater Overall Health Of All The Systems, Including The Nerves

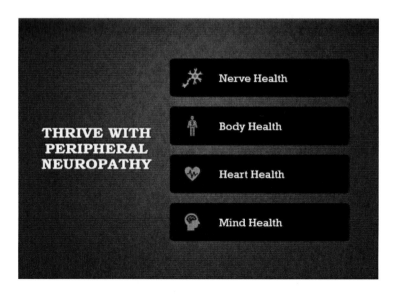

The medical term *Failure to Thrive* is utilized in early childhood development to describe an infant that fails to grow or gain weight as expected. In older individuals, the geriatric population, a similar term is utilized to describe an older individual that is in decline in ability, skill and even weight. If the older individual is worsening more quickly than expected this term is often used.

With that definition of *Thrive*, if an individual is able to function as expected without the discomfort, distraction and disability of peripheral neuropathy it would be considered a success. My opinion, however, is this is too small a goal to work towards. Instead, I want you to truly *Thrive*, meaning grow, progress and increase you influence and impact on the world. To truly *Thrive* you should be living and extraordinary life even better than you could hope.

Before you can step into that *Extraordinary Life,* however, you must first improve your overall health. For purposes of *Thriving With Peripheral Neuropathy*, I break health into four distinct categories that we will discuss here.

Nerve Health

When it comes to *Thriving With Peripheral Neuropathy,* it is imperative that you start with nerve health. In fact, this book has been an entire framework for treating, improving, and optimizing nerve health. The four pillars of nerve health are:

1. **Understand Peripheral Neuropathy** (including your unique personal neuropathy presentation)
2. **Manage The Symptoms of Neuropathy**
3. **Control Nerve Damage**
4. **Thrive with Peripheral Neuropathy**

NERVE HEALTH

2. MANAGE
The Symptoms of Neuropathy

1. UNDERSTAND
Peripheral Neuropathy Personally

4. THRIVE
With Peripheral Neuropathy

3. CONTROL
Nerve Damage

As you carefully implement the teaching in this book, you will lay the initial foundation for true health and give yourself the best chance to truly *THRIVE*.

Body Health

The other aspect of health discussed throughout this book is body health. I, however, want to take this further and include both physical and emotional health. The true definition of *Thrive* requires both these aspects of health as well.

- *Physical Health* – To be physically healthy you must optimize all aspects of health:
    - o Proper nutrition – how you eat including both foods and supplementation as needed.
    - o Regular exercise – usually at least 30 minutes 5 times a day.
    - o Sufficient sleep – as discussed earlier in this book most individuals require 7-8 hours of good sleep (restful sleep).
    - o Abundant hydration – remember the water!
    - o Health social interactions – this is important! *(see heart health below)*
- *Emotional Health* – This aspect of health involves learning to find joy and happiness in life. Although I don't have space to go into great depth on how to be happy, I want to introduce the concept of *Eudeamonic Happiness.* I was taught this principle through Transformational Academy by Joeel & Natalie Rivera. I then modified this to what I am teaching below.

    The most common form of what we call happiness is *Hedonistic Happiness.* This is happiness influenced by the outside world and often leads to seeking pleasure and avoiding discomfort to find happiness. This is giving away power to your external environment where "Happiness happens to you." This is a limited happiness that is often fleeting because it is dependent on everything going well.

Eudeamonic Happiness is purpose based or internally based. This signifies you *BECOMING HAPPY* or in other words you ARE happy at the core. This takes all power away from external forces because your happiness comes from you not what is happening to you. There are 6 steps to this type of happiness and is learned: *(HAPPY Mood)*

- o HUNGER – The first step is based on desire. We find our happiness by fulfilling our needs. If our needs aren't being met, this is the first step to moving from hedonistic to eudeamonic happiness.
- o ACCEPTANCE – The next step is learning to recognize who we are and accepting the fact that we are Extraordinary and deserve to Live an Extraordinary life (deserve to be happy). This is based on overcoming any limiting beliefs or self-doubt.
- o PERSONALITY – The next logical step is starting to understand your identity. Your understanding of who you are, including your strengths, talents and weaknesses can help you start to move toward "being" happy even in your limitations. Often this level is still very externally based because our identity is often influences deeply by external input.

o PERCEPTION – Often our reality is based on perception, either from past experiences or possible future experiences. When we overcome perception and realize we can be happy now no matter what is happening, we take a huge step towards eudeamonic happiness.

o YOU – The next step is where the switch truly starts to happen. This utilizes the idea of neuroplasticity (ability to rewire the brain) to truly understand who you are and step into that role. As you recognize your strengths, talents and weaknesses you have greater power to live the life you deserve. This leads to greater intrinsic or eudeamonic happiness.

o MOOD – The final step is utilizing two powerful tools to "choose" happiness.

- *Joy* – Through looking for the blessing or benefits of every situation, every interaction, you start to find joy in all aspects of life.

- *Gratitude* – I can't underemphasize the power of gratitude. This is one of the quickest ways to step into eudeamonic happiness.

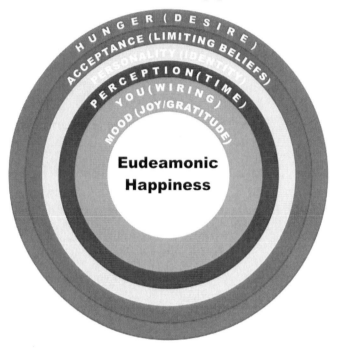

Heart Health

For heart health here I am not talking about the physical heart (that is covered under *Body Health*). Instead, I am talking about two important aspects of overall health: *Social Health* and *Spiritual Health.*

- *Social Health* – One of the most powerful tools for health is both your social interactions with others and your relationships. Studies show improved health when you have a healthy social life.

    For example, a happy marriage leads to greater health and fewer physical problems. The opposite is also true. But did you know that life is also considered more fulfilling and enjoyable? Doesn't that help you understand how this aspect will help you *Thrive?*

    There are several methods to improve Social Health:
    - *Surround Yourself With People That Make You Better.* Jim Rohn taught, "You're the average of the five people you spend you spend the most time with." You want to surround yourself with people that help you *Thrive.*
    - *Go All In!* A successful, fulfilling and rewarding relationship is the relationship in which you both *go all in.* Are you willing to give it your all?
    - *Serve With All Your Heart.* Don't underestimate the healing power of service. If you truly love others and serve them, you will be blessed with individuals that love you. There is power in that supporting love!
- *Spiritual Health* – Although there is some overlap, I am going to invite you to allow God into your life.

I am not going to apologize (you can use your own definition of God, but I know Who I mean) for using this term. There are actually scientific studies showing power in the faith that comes through believing in God. There are even proven studies on the benefits of prayer (personal and even by an unknown individual) when managing peripheral neuropathy.

I invite you to access the power that comes through personal prayer, belief in God and faith that He desires you to *Thrive* in this life. *I know this to be true!*

Mind Health

There is amazing power in the mind! The current studies of how you think, how you believe can be called mindset or mindfulness. Really what it comes down to is the simple quote by Henry Ford, *"Whether you think you CAN or you think you CAN'T, you're right!"* So where is your mind?

So one of the key pieces to *Thriving* in this life is improving the health of your mind. Let me give you four daily steps to improve your mindset:

1. *Begin and End Each Day With Gratitude* (this will not be discussed here as it is discussed in depth in Chapter 9)

2. *Own The Stage That Is Your Mind* – Each of us have a stage, our mind, that is constantly being bombarded by acts, commercials and side shows. Everyone wants time on the stage of your mind. It is your job to be the stage manager and director to ensure only what you want entering your mind has access. Eliminate anything and

everything that will interfere with the growth and positive mindset you desire. *(For example, some individuals have eliminated social media, others limit news, and still others search for uplifting and positive influences only from the internet. It is your mind, so it is your choice!)*

One powerful aspect of controlling your stage is not giving anyone the power to decide your mood. As we discussed earlier in this book nobody can make you sad, mad or even happy without your permission. Decide each day how the day will go and don't give anyone or anything the power to change that resolve. You can completely control HOW you react to the day and what others say or do to you.

3. *A Healthy Body Produces A Healthy Mind* – Ensure you participate in healthy eating, regular exercise and appropriate sleep to ensure your body is working at the highest level. Studies show the mind is more clear, neurons of the brain more active and thought patterns more integrated. Your mind is only as good as the nutrients or nutrition you feed it. Why not feed it the nutrients and nutrition of a genius so it can help you *reach your goals, live your dream and enjoy and extraordinary life?*

4. *The Power of Meditation* – The term meditation makes many individuals uncomfortable. If you would prefer, you can call it mindfulness. Whatever you call it, it is an opportunity to unify the body and mind in such a way that you can step into the power of peak performance throughout the day. Let me explain the two methods I use each day:

a. *Prayer* – Daily prayer (often multiple times a day) has become an important part of my life. I use it to talk to God, but it also provides me a focus and a method to recognize all the blessings I have. *At one time I thought it was all I needed for mindfulness, but that is no longer true.*

b. *Meditation* – I try to spend at least 3-5 minutes each day in focused meditation (sometimes it is longer, but I am still learning to do this well). The most effective method for me is to focus on visualizing me accomplishing my goals, living the life I want to live and feeling the emotion and pride that comes with that. This often provides me the insights I need to make the appropriate steps to move toward that life.

LIVE AN EXTRAORDINARY LIFE EVEN WITH PERIPHERAL NEUROPATHY

Your Greatest Resource To Overcoming Neuropathy Is You!

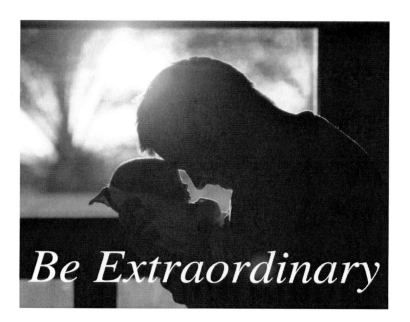

I lifted that small 6lb 1oz baby girl from my wife's arms and looked into those beautiful blue eyes. She was perfect! As I felt her in my arms, I started getting overwhelmed! Could I be the father she deserves? Could I help her realize that even with her weaknesses or perceived flaws she was much more than normal, average or ordinary? Could I help her realize that she truly is extraordinary? Could I help her step into that extraordinary so that she could live the life she was born to live? That has been one of my life missions as each of my 11 children came into this world, I had the same thoughts, the same concerns and ultimately the same resolve to give them that gift.

I have the same desire for you! Do you realize that you are extraordinary? There is nobody just like you! Nobody has your strengths, your talents and even your weaknesses. Because of that nobody can have the influence and impact on the world that you can. For this reason, I need you! In fact, the world needs you to live that "Extraordinary Life" you were born to live. That is my goal for this book, my goal for each and every individual I meet (with or without peripheral neuropathy). I hope you have recognized that I have given you the foundation that will make this possible. Through the rest of this chapter, I will help you recognize what that can and should look like. Are your ready to *Be Extraordinary*?

Define Extraordinary

The biggest question I am asked when I talk about *Being Extraordinary* is, "What does it mean to Be Extraordinary or Live an Extraordinary Life?" The truth is I can't answer that for you. Extraordinary is an individual definition. Instead, I will ask you several questions to help you create your own definition. This will be your goal for managing peripheral neuropathy.

- What would you be doing if you didn't have peripheral neuropathy? What is it keeping you from doing that you want to be?
- If you had no limitations (not physical, not health, and possibly even not financial), what would your life look like?
- As you look at everything in your life, what would you like to spend more time doing or who would you like to spend more time with?
- If you got to observe your funeral, what would you want people to say about you? (What would it take to BECOME that individual?)

As you work on answering these questions, think deeply, include what it would look like, what it would feel like, what emotions you would have if it were true. The more real you make this definition, the more likely your subconscious mind can start working on helping it become a reality. This will also give you the vision you can think about during your daily meditation sessions.

Build Extraordinary

Once you know what *Extraordinary* looks like for you, it is time to build it. Start creating the daily habits that will provide the foundation for this new life. More importantly, start working each day to make it a reality. The final question earlier in this chapter talks about "What would it take to BECOME?" It is those steps you want to take.

Let me teach you a powerful principle of goal setting. You have probably heard about SMART goals, but I have modified several to ensure you set goals without limiting your ability to achieve. For our purposes SMART is as follows:

- **S – Specific**: It is important that it be clear, concise and focused. You must have something to work towards.
- **M – Measurable**: Must be trackable or able to be measured. How will you know you got the results?
- **A – Actionable**: The goal must be under your control. Can you influence the results? If you can't the goal is wrong. *(Often A is used for attainable, but that causes you to limit the possibilities.)*
- **R – Relevant**: This ensures the goal is in accordance with your vision, your Extraordinary. If it isn't helping you move towards that goal, again it is the wrong goal. *(Often R is used for realistic, but this also limits the possibilities.)*
- **T – Timebound**: There must be a deadline. As you get closer to the deadline the possibility of reaching the goal goes up.

Through this process of SMART goals, you can create a process to build your Extraordinary Life. You begin with your vision of what *Extraordinary* looks like. Create high hard goals that lead you to that vision and then create daily goals that lead to each high hard goal. This is a powerful process that can be repeated for any Transformative Major Purpose – in this case Becoming Extraordinary and Living an Extraordinary Life.

S — Specific

- Be Clear and Precise
- Focused and Narrow
- Identify an Exact Outcome

M — Measurable

- Make Trackable
- Make Quatifiable
- Ensure Identifiable Progress

A — Actionable

- Can You Influence The Results?
- Within Your Locus of Control

R — Relevant

- Aligned With Your Values
- Built On Your Major Purpose

T — Timebound

- Set A Deadline
- Be Specific On The Timeframe
- When Exactly Will It Be Done?

Live Extraordinary

Once you have set your goals to *Build Extraordinary*, it is time to start living in accordance with these goals. Start living the extraordinary life. Through this process you will start to find the HOW. This will occur through a more active RAS filter that is looking for all the ways the *Extraordinary Life* can become an active part of your life.

The Power of Gratitude

The most effective way to speed this process is through the power of gratitude. You may not realize but gratitude is a powerful stimulant of happiness and joy, but also helps you access peak performance in your daily life. Let me give you three simple steps to access this power:

- **Morning Gratitude:** One powerful technique to start you day with gratitude is to name three things you are grateful for first thing in the morning. This can be done through morning prayer, or you can create a *Gratitude Journal* and write down these three things. By starting your day with gratitude, typically the entire day will go better.

- **Recognize Blessings:** The next step is to go throughout the day looking for blessing, for things that you can be grateful for. As we discussed earlier, what you focus on the brain will help you recognize (remember the RAS filter).

- **Nightly Gratitude:** The final step is to write (physically write as there are studies showing a greater benefit to handwritten responses) at least one thing that happened that day that you are grateful for.

Don't underestimate this practice of ending your day in gratitude!

This Is A Lifetime Pursuit

The final step to *Living An Extraordinary Life* is the understanding that it is a constant pursuit. You will need to work every moment of every day to ensure continued *Extraordinary* or you will slip back into normal, average and ordinary. The world is constantly pushing you towards the status quo and only if you are actively working at it will you reach the life you desire, the life you deserve!

Remember, my goal for you is to Reach Your Goals, Live Your Dream and Enjoy An Extraordinary Life...even with Peripheral Neuropathy. You deserve it!

NOTES

- Barrell K, Smith AG. Peripheral Neuropathy. Med Clin North Am. 2019 Mar;103(2):383-397. doi: 10.1016/j.mcna.2018.10.006. Epub 2018 Dec 17. PMID: 30704689.
- Siao P, Kaku M. A Clinician's Approach to Peripheral Neuropathy. Semin Neurol. 2019 Oct;39(5):519-530. doi: 10.1055/s-0039-1694747. Epub 2019 Oct 22. PMID: 31639835.
- Watson JC, Dyck PJ. Peripheral Neuropathy: A Practical Approach to Diagnosis and Symptom Management. Mayo Clin Proc. 2015 Jul;90(7):940-51. doi: 10.1016/j.mayocp.2015.05.004. PMID: 26141332.
- Freeman R. Autonomic Peripheral Neuropathy. Continuum (Minneap Minn). 2020 Feb;26(1):58-71. doi: 10.1212/CON.0000000000000825. PMID: 31996622.
- Castelli G, Desai KM, Cantone RE. Peripheral Neuropathy: Evaluation and Differential Diagnosis. Am Fam Physician. 2020 Dec 15;102(12):732-739. PMID: 33320513.
- Nold CS, Nozaki K. Peripheral neuropathy: Clinical pearls for making the diagnosis. JAAPA. 2020 Jan;33(1):9-15. doi: 10.1097/01.JAA.0000615460.45150.e0. Erratum in: JAAPA. 2020 Feb;33(2):1-3. PMID: 31880643.
- Ben-Horin I, Kahan P, Ryvo L, Inbar M, Lev-Ari S, Geva R. Acupuncture and Reflexology for Chemotherapy-Induced Peripheral Neuropathy in Breast Cancer. Integr Cancer Ther. 2017 Sep;16(3):258-262. doi: 10.1177/1534735417690254. Epub 2017 Feb 2. PMID: 28150504; PMCID: PMC5759933.
- Haryani H, Fetzer SJ, Wu CL, Hsu YY. Chemotherapy-Induced Peripheral Neuropathy Assessment Tools: A Systematic Review. Oncol Nurs Forum. 2017 May 1;44(3):E111-E123. doi: 10.1188/17.ONF.E111-E123. PMID: 28635977.
- Katona I, Weis J. Diseases of the peripheral nerves. Handb Clin Neurol. 2017;145:453-474. doi: 10.1016/B978-0-12-802395-2.00031-6. PMID: 28987189.
- England JD, Asbury AK. Peripheral neuropathy. Lancet. 2004 Jun 26;363(9427):2151-61. doi: 10.1016/S0140-6736(04)16508-2. PMID: 15220040.
- Dive D, Lievens I, Moonen G, Wang FC. La neuropathie diabétique périphérique [Diabetic peripheral neuropathy]. Rev Med Liege. 2005 May-Jun;60(5-6):490-7. French. PMID: 16035316.

- Ugalde V, Rosen BS. Ischemic peripheral neuropathy. Phys Med Rehabil Clin N Am. 2001 May;12(2):365-80. PMID: 11345013.
- Hughes RA. Peripheral neuropathy. BMJ. 2002 Feb 23;324(7335):466-9. doi: 10.1136/bmj.324.7335.466. PMID: 11859051; PMCID: PMC1122393.
- Craig AS, Richardson JK. Acquired peripheral neuropathy. Phys Med Rehabil Clin N Am. 2003 May;14(2):365-86. doi: 10.1016/s1047-9651(02)00118-3. PMID: 12795521.
- García-Cabo C, Morís G. Peripheral neuropathy: an underreported neurologic manifestation of inflammatory bowel disease. Eur J Intern Med. 2015 Sep;26(7):468-75. doi: 10.1016/j.ejim.2015.07.013. Epub 2015 Jul 23. PMID: 26211733.
- Jones MR, Urits I, Wolf J, Corrigan D, Colburn L, Peterson E, Williamson A, Viswanath O. Drug-Induced Peripheral Neuropathy: A Narrative Review. Curr Clin Pharmacol. 2020;15(1):38-48. doi: 10.2174/1574884714666190121154813. PMID: 30666914; PMCID: PMC7365998.
- Vilholm OJ, Christensen AA, Zedan AH, Itani M. Drug-induced peripheral neuropathy. Basic Clin Pharmacol Toxicol. 2014 Aug;115(2):185-92. doi: 10.1111/bcpt.12261. Epub 2014 May 20. PMID: 24786912.
- Seretny M, Currie GL, Sena ES, Ramnarine S, Grant R, MacLeod MR, Colvin LA, Fallon M. Incidence, prevalence, and predictors of chemotherapy-induced peripheral neuropathy: A systematic review and meta-analysis. Pain. 2014 Dec;155(12):2461-2470. doi: 10.1016/j.pain.2014.09.020. Epub 2014 Sep 23. PMID: 25261162.
- Delanian S, Lefaix JL, Pradat PF. Radiation-induced neuropathy in cancer survivors. Radiother Oncol. 2012 Dec;105(3):273-82. doi: 10.1016/j.radonc.2012.10.012. PMID: 23245644.
- Melzack, Ronald (1990). "Phantom limbs and the concept of a neuromatrix". *Trends in Neurosciences*. **13** (3): 88–92. doi:10.1016/0166-2236(90)90179-E. PMID 1691874. S2CID 8639462.
- Melzack R. From the gate to the neuromatrix. Pain. 1999 Aug;Suppl 6:S121-S126. doi: 10.1016/S0304-3959(99)00145-1. PMID: 10491980.
- Olney RK. Neuropathies associated with connective tissue disease. Semin Neurol. 1998;18(1):63-72. doi: 10.1055/s-2008-1040862. PMID: 9562668.
- Scherer SS. Finding the Causes of Inherited Neuropathies. *Arch Neurol.* 2006;63(6):812–816. doi:10.1001/archneur.63.6.812
- Khamseh, Mohammad & kazemi khoo, Nooshafarin & Aghili, Rokhsareh & Forogh, Bijan & M. Lajevardi & Dabaghian, Fataneh & A, Goushegir & Malek, Mojtaba. (2011). Diabetic distal symmetric polyneuropathy: effect of low-intensity laser therapy.. Lasers in Medical Science. 26. 831.

- Gwathmey KG, Grogan J. Nutritional neuropathies. Muscle Nerve. 2020 Jul;62(1):13-29. doi: 10.1002/mus.26783. Epub 2019 Dec 26. PMID: 31837157.

- Jennaro TS, Fang F, Kidwell KM, Smith EML, Vangipuram K, Burness ML, Griggs JJ, Van Poznak C, Hayes DF, Henry NL, Hertz DL. Vitamin D deficiency increases severity of paclitaxel-induced peripheral neuropathy. Breast Cancer Res Treat. 2020 Apr;180(3):707-714. doi: 10.1007/s10549-020-05584-8. Epub 2020 Mar 12. PMID: 32166478; PMCID: PMC7945004.

- Ahmed MA, Muntingh G, Rheeder P. Vitamin B12 deficiency in metformin-treated type-2 diabetes patients, prevalence and association with peripheral neuropathy. BMC Pharmacol Toxicol. 2016 Oct 7;17(1):44. doi: 10.1186/s40360-016-0088-3. PMID: 27716423; PMCID: PMC5054613.

- Jayabalan B, Low LL. Vitamin B supplementation for diabetic peripheral neuropathy. Singapore Med J. 2016 Feb;57(2):55-9. doi: 10.11622/smedj.2016027. PMID: 26892473; PMCID: PMC4759374.

- Shible AA, Ramadurai D, Gergen D, Reynolds PM. Dry Beriberi Due to Thiamine Deficiency Associated with Peripheral Neuropathy and Wernicke's Encephalopathy Mimicking Guillain-Barré syndrome: A Case Report and Review of the Literature. Am J Case Rep. 2019 Mar 13;20:330-334. doi: 10.12659/AJCR.914051. PMID: 30862772; PMCID: PMC6429982.

- Staff NP, Windebank AJ. Peripheral neuropathy due to vitamin deficiency, toxins, and medications. Continuum (Minneap Minn). 2014 Oct;20(5 Peripheral Nervous System Disorders):1293-306. doi: 10.1212/01.CON.0000455880.06675.5a. PMID: 25299283; PMCID: PMC4208100.

- Alharbi TJ, Tourkmani AM, Abdelhay O, Alkhashan HI, Al-Asmari AK, Bin Rsheed AM, Abuhaimed SN, Mohammed N, AlRasheed AN, AlHarbi NG. The association of metformin use with vitamin B12 deficiency and peripheral neuropathy in Saudi individuals with type 2 diabetes mellitus. PLoS One. 2018 Oct 15;13(10):e0204420. doi: 10.1371/journal.pone.0204420. PMID: 30321183; PMCID: PMC6188756.

- Maiya RP, Messing RO. Peripheral systems: neuropathy. Handb Clin Neurol. 2014;125:513-25. doi: 10.1016/B978-0-444-62619-6.00029-X. PMID: 25307593.

- Putz Z, Martos T, Németh N, Körei AE, Szabó M, Vági OE, Kempler MS, Kempler P. D-vitamin és neuropathia [Vitamin D and neuropathy]. Orv Hetil. 2013 Dec 22;154(51):2012-5. Hungarian. doi: 10.1556/OH.2013.29769. PMID: 24334132.

- Fenton BW, Shih E, Zolton J. The neurobiology of pain perception in normal and persistent pain. Pain Manag. 2015;5(4):297-317. doi: 10.2217/pmt.15.27. Epub 2015 Jun 19. PMID: 26088531.

- Cárdenas Fernández R. La neuromatrix y su importancia en la neurobiologia del dolor [The neuromatrix and its importance in pain neurobiology]. Invest Clin. 2015 Jun;56(2):109-10. Spanish. PMID: 26299052.

- Clijsen R, Brunner A, Barbero M, Clarys P, Taeymans J. Effects of low-level laser therapy on pain in patients with musculoskeletal disorders: a systematic review and meta-analysis. Eur J Phys Rehabil Med. 2017 Aug;53(4):603-610. doi: 10.23736/S1973-9087.17.04432-X. Epub 2017 Jan 30. PMID: 28145397.

- Clijsen R, Brunner A, Barbero M, Clarys P, Taeymans J. Effects of low-level laser therapy on pain in patients with musculoskeletal disorders: a systematic review and meta-analysis. Eur J Phys Rehabil Med. 2017 Aug;53(4):603-610. doi: 10.23736/S1973-9087.17.04432-X. Epub 2017 Jan 30. PMID: 28145397.

- Mussttaf RA, Jenkins DFL, Jha AN. Assessing the impact of low level laser therapy (LLLT) on biological systems: a review. Int J Radiat Biol. 2019 Feb;95(2):120-143. doi: 10.1080/09553002.2019.1524944. Epub 2019 Jan 7. PMID: 30614743.

- M A, Ummer V S, Maiya AG, Hande M. Low level laser therapy for the patients with painful diabetic peripheral neuropathy - A systematic review. Diabetes Metab Syndr. 2019 Jul-Aug;13(4):2667-2670. doi: 10.1016/j.dsx.2019.07.035. Epub 2019 Jul 13. PMID: 31405692.

- Abdel-Wahhab KG, Daoud EM, El Gendy A, Mourad HH, Mannaa FA, Saber MM. Efficiencies of Low-Level Laser Therapy (LLLT) and Gabapentin in the Management of Peripheral Neuropathy: Diabetic Neuropathy. Appl Biochem Biotechnol. 2018 Sep;186(1):161-173. doi: 10.1007/s12010-018-2729-z. Epub 2018 Mar 12. PMID: 29527628.

- Fallah A, Mirzaei A, Gutknecht N, Demneh AS. Clinical effectiveness of low-level laser treatment on peripheral somatosensory neuropathy. Lasers Med Sci. 2017 Apr;32(3):721-728. doi: 10.1007/s10103-016-2137-y. Epub 2017 Jan 10. PMID: 28074305.

- Çakici N, Fakkel TM, van Neck JW, Verhagen AP, Coert JH. Systematic review of treatments for diabetic peripheral neuropathy. Diabet Med. 2016 Nov;33(11):1466-1476. doi: 10.1111/dme.13083. Epub 2016 Feb 21. PMID: 26822889.

- Xu L, Zhang Y, Huang Y. Advances in the Treatment of Neuropathic Pain. Adv Exp Med Biol. 2016;904:117-29. doi: 10.1007/978-94-017-7537-3_9. PMID: 26900067.

- Bartkoski S, Day M. Alpha-Lipoic Acid for Treatment of Diabetic Peripheral Neuropathy. Am Fam Physician. 2016 May 1;93(9):786. PMID: 27175957.

- Carozzi VA, Canta A, Chiorazzi A. Chemotherapy-induced peripheral neuropathy: What do we know about mechanisms? Neurosci Lett. 2015 Jun 2;596:90-107. doi: 10.1016/j.neulet.2014.10.014.

Epub 2014 Oct 22. Erratum in: Neurosci Lett. 2015 Jun 2;596():108. PMID: 25459280.

- Schapira AH. Mitochondrial diseases. Lancet. 2012 May 12;379(9828):1825-34. doi: 10.1016/S0140-6736(11)61305-6. Epub 2012 Apr 5. PMID: 22482939.
- Persson AK, Hoeijmakers JGJ, Estacion M, Black JA, Waxman SG. Sodium Channels, Mitochondria, and Axonal Degeneration in Peripheral Neuropathy. Trends Mol Med. 2016 May;22(5):377-390. doi: 10.1016/j.molmed.2016.03.008. Epub 2016 Apr 13. PMID: 27085813.
- Trecarichi A, Flatters SJL. Mitochondrial dysfunction in the pathogenesis of chemotherapy-induced peripheral neuropathy. Int Rev Neurobiol. 2019;145:83-126. doi: 10.1016/bs.irn.2019.05.001. Epub 2019 Jun 6. PMID: 31208528.
- Trecarichi A, Flatters SJL. Mitochondrial dysfunction in the pathogenesis of chemotherapy-induced peripheral neuropathy. Int Rev Neurobiol. 2019;145:83-126. doi: 10.1016/bs.irn.2019.05.001. Epub 2019 Jun 6. PMID: 31208528.
- Singleton JR, Smith AG, Marcus RL. Exercise as Therapy for Diabetic and Prediabetic Neuropathy. Curr Diab Rep. 2015 Dec;15(12):120. doi: 10.1007/s11892-015-0682-6. PMID: 26538074.
- Singleton JR, Smith AG, Marcus RL. Exercise as Therapy for Diabetic and Prediabetic Neuropathy. Curr Diab Rep. 2015 Dec;15(12):120. doi: 10.1007/s11892-015-0682-6. PMID: 26538074.
- Kluding PM, Pasnoor M, Singh R, Jernigan S, Farmer K, Rucker J, Sharma NK, Wright DE. The effect of exercise on neuropathic symptoms, nerve function, and cutaneous innervation in people with diabetic peripheral neuropathy. J Diabetes Complications. 2012 Sep-Oct;26(5):424-9. doi: 10.1016/j.jdiacomp.2012.05.007. Epub 2012 Jun 18. PMID: 22717465; PMCID: PMC3436981.
- Rowin J. Integrative neuromuscular medicine: Neuropathy and neuropathic pain: Consider the alternatives. Muscle Nerve. 2019 Aug;60(2):124-136. doi: 10.1002/mus.26510. Epub 2019 May 30. PMID: 31074875.
- Memme JM, Erlich AT, Phukan G, Hood DA. Exercise and mitochondrial health. J Physiol. 2021 Feb;599(3):803-817. doi: 10.1113/JP278853. Epub 2019 Dec 9. PMID: 31674658.
- Bernardo TC, Marques-Aleixo I, Beleza J, Oliveira PJ, Ascensão A, Magalhães J. Physical Exercise and Brain Mitochondrial Fitness: The Possible Role Against Alzheimer's Disease. Brain Pathol. 2016 Sep;26(5):648-63. doi: 10.1111/bpa.12403. PMID: 27328058; PMCID: PMC8029062.
- Bishop DJ, Botella J, Genders AJ, Lee MJ, Saner NJ, Kuang J, Yan X, Granata C. High-Intensity Exercise and Mitochondrial Biogenesis: Current Controversies and Future Research Directions.

Physiology (Bethesda). 2019 Jan 1;34(1):56-70. doi: 10.1152/physiol.00038.2018. PMID: 30540234.

- Freeman R. Autonomic Peripheral Neuropathy. Continuum (Minneap Minn). 2020 Feb;26(1):58-71. doi: 10.1212/CON.0000000000000825. PMID: 31996622.

- Zaeem Z, Siddiqi ZA, Zochodne DW. Autonomic involvement in Guillain-Barré syndrome: an update. Clin Auton Res. 2019 Jun;29(3):289-299. doi: 10.1007/s10286-018-0542-y. Epub 2018 Jul 17. PMID: 30019292.

- Kaur D, Tiwana H, Stino A, Sandroni P. Autonomic neuropathies. Muscle Nerve. 2021 Jan;63(1):10-21. doi: 10.1002/mus.27048. Epub 2020 Sep 14. PMID: 32926436.

- Zhou L. Small Fiber Neuropathy. Semin Neurol. 2019 Oct;39(5):570-577. doi: 10.1055/s-0039-1688977. Epub 2019 Oct 22. PMID: 31639840.

- Sène D. Small fiber neuropathy: Diagnosis, causes, and treatment. Joint Bone Spine. 2018 Oct;85(5):553-559. doi: 10.1016/j.jbspin.2017.11.002. Epub 2017 Nov 16. PMID: 29154979.

- Sopacua M, Hoeijmakers JGJ, Merkies ISJ, Lauria G, Waxman SG, Faber CG. Small-fiber neuropathy: Expanding the clinical pain universe. J Peripher Nerv Syst. 2019 Mar;24(1):19-33. doi: 10.1111/jns.12298. Epub 2019 Jan 8. PMID: 30569495.

- Saperstein DS. Small Fiber Neuropathy. Neurol Clin. 2020 Aug;38(3):607-618. doi: 10.1016/j.ncl.2020.04.001. PMID: 32703472.

- Zeidman LA. Advances in the Management of Small Fiber Neuropathy. Neurol Clin. 2021 Feb;39(1):113-131. doi: 10.1016/j.ncl.2020.09.006. Epub 2020 Nov 7. PMID: 33223078.

- Martínez-Lavín M. Fibromyalgia and small fiber neuropathy: the plot thickens! Clin Rheumatol. 2018 Dec;37(12):3167-3171. doi: 10.1007/s10067-018-4300-2. Epub 2018 Sep 20. PMID: 30238382.

- Siedler G, Sommer C, Üçeyler N. Pain-related evoked potentials in patients with large, mixed, and small fiber neuropathy. Clin Neurophysiol. 2020 Mar;131(3):635-641. doi: 10.1016/j.clinph.2019.12.006. Epub 2019 Dec 26. PMID: 31978848.

- Haroutounian S, Todorovic MS, Leinders M, Campagnolo M, Gewandter JS, Dworkin RH, Freeman R. Diagnostic criteria for idiopathic small fiber neuropathy: A systematic review. Muscle Nerve. 2021 Feb;63(2):170-177. doi: 10.1002/mus.27070. Epub 2020 Sep 29. PMID: 32989823.

- Gomatos EL, Rehman A. Sensory Neuropathy. 2021 Jul 11. In: StatPearls [Internet]. Treasure Island (FL): StatPearls Publishing; 2021 Jan–. PMID: 32644446.

- Tomiyama M, Yagihashi S. [Neuropathy and unmyelinated epidermal nerve fibers]. Brain Nerve. 2012 Nov;64(11):1225-31. Japanese. PMID: 23131732.
- Dellon AL. Abnormal skin biopsy for intraepidermal nerve fibers: When "Decreased small nerve fibers" is not "Small fiber neuropathy". Microsurgery. 2015 Oct;35(7):505-6. doi: 10.1002/micr.22372. Epub 2015 Jan 6. PMID: 25565414.
- Hussain N, Said ASA. Mindfulness-Based Meditation Versus Progressive Relaxation Meditation: Impact on Chronic Pain in Older Female Patients With Diabetic Neuropathy. J Evid Based Integr Med. 2019 Jan-Dec;24:2515690X19876599. doi: 10.1177/2515690X19876599. PMID: 31544476; PMCID: PMC6757487.
- Baute V, Zelnik D, Curtis J, Sadeghifar F. Complementary and Alternative Medicine for Painful Peripheral Neuropathy. Curr Treat Options Neurol. 2019 Sep 2;21(9):44. doi: 10.1007/s11940-019-0584-z. PMID: 31478093.
- Brami C, Bao T, Deng G. Natural products and complementary therapies for chemotherapy-induced peripheral neuropathy: A systematic review. Crit Rev Oncol Hematol. 2016 Feb;98:325-34. doi: 10.1016/j.critrevonc.2015.11.014. Epub 2015 Nov 23. PMID: 26652982; PMCID: PMC4727999.
- Galantino ML, Tiger R, Brooks J, Jang S, Wilson K. Impact of Somatic Yoga and Meditation on Fall Risk, Function, and Quality of Life for Chemotherapy-Induced Peripheral Neuropathy Syndrome in Cancer Survivors. Integr Cancer Ther. 2019 Jan-Dec;18:1534735419850627. doi: 10.1177/1534735419850627. PMID: 31131640; PMCID: PMC6537287.
- van Laake-Geelen CCM, Smeets RJEM, Quadflieg SPAB, Kleijnen J, Verbunt JA. The effect of exercise therapy combined with psychological therapy on physical activity and quality of life in patients with painful diabetic neuropathy: a systematic review. Scand J Pain. 2019 Jul 26;19(3):433-439. doi: 10.1515/sjpain-2019-0001. PMID: 31112511.
- Manji H. Toxic neuropathy. Curr Opin Neurol. 2011 Oct;24(5):484-90. doi: 10.1097/WCO.0b013e32834a94b6. PMID: 21897232.
- Jortner BS. Nerve Fiber Regeneration in Toxic Peripheral Neuropathy. Toxicol Pathol. 2020 Jan;48(1):144-151. doi: 10.1177/0192623319854089. Epub 2019 Jun 11. PMID: 31184283.
- Dervaux A, Laqueille X. Le traitement par thiamine (vitamine B1) dans l'alcoolodépendance [Thiamine (vitamin B1) treatment in patients with alcohol dependence]. Presse Med. 2017 Mar;46(2 Pt 1):165-171. French. doi: 10.1016/j.lpm.2016.07.025. Epub 2016 Nov 3. PMID: 27818067.

- Wiley KD, Gupta M. Vitamin B1 Thiamine Deficiency. 2021 Jun 21. In: StatPearls [Internet]. Treasure Island (FL): StatPearls Publishing; 2021 Jan–. PMID: 30725889.

- Chopra K, Tiwari V. Alcoholic neuropathy: possible mechanisms and future treatment possibilities. Br J Clin Pharmacol. 2012 Mar;73(3):348-62. doi: 10.1111/j.1365-2125.2011.04111.x. PMID: 21988193; PMCID: PMC3370340.

- Almoznino G, Benoliel R, Sharav Y, Haviv Y. Sleep disorders and chronic craniofacial pain: Characteristics and management possibilities. Sleep Med Rev. 2017 Jun;33:39-50. doi: 10.1016/j.smrv.2016.04.005. Epub 2016 May 11. PMID: 27321865.

- Choi D, Kim BY, Jung CH, Kim CH, Mok JO. Association between Sleep Quality and Painless Diabetic Peripheral Neuropathy Assessed by Current Perception Threshold in Type 2 Diabetes Mellitus. Diabetes Metab J. 2021 May;45(3):358-367. doi: 10.4093/dmj.2019.0219. Epub 2020 Aug 6. PMID: 32794384; PMCID: PMC8164947.

- Simpson NS, Gibbs EL, Matheson GO. Optimizing sleep to maximize performance: implications and recommendations for elite athletes. Scand J Med Sci Sports. 2017 Mar;27(3):266-274. doi: 10.1111/sms.12703. Epub 2016 Jul 1. PMID: 27367265.

- Reutrakul S, Van Cauter E. Sleep influences on obesity, insulin resistance, and risk of type 2 diabetes. Metabolism. 2018 Jul;84:56-66. doi: 10.1016/j.metabol.2018.02.010. Epub 2018 Mar 3. PMID: 29510179.

- Sampasa-Kanyinga H, Colman I, Goldfield GS, Janssen I, Wang J, Podinic I, Tremblay MS, Saunders TJ, Sampson M, Chaput JP. Combinations of physical activity, sedentary time, and sleep duration and their associations with depressive symptoms and other mental health problems in children and adolescents: a systematic review. Int J Behav Nutr Phys Act. 2020 Jun 5;17(1):72. doi: 10.1186/s12966-020-00976-x. PMID: 32503638; PMCID: PMC7273653.

ABOUT THE AUTHOR

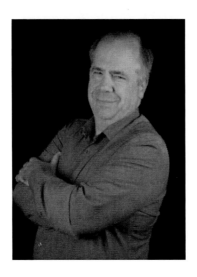

Dr Brandt R Gibson is the father of 11 children, 2 bonus children (that married two of his children), grandfather to 1 (so far) and husband of an amazing woman, the three roles he enjoys the most. He is also a podiatric physician (specializing in foot and ankle care) and has revolutionized the care of Peripheral Neuropathy for his patients. He also thrives on service to his community, state and his church, including serving a church mission to Brazil for two years, coaching many soccer teams over the years and previously working in the Boy Scouts of America for over 24 years.

Dr Gibson is as physician, author, coach and speaker who empowers individuals to Be Extraordinary by Becoming Concordant in their strengths, talents and weaknesses and Unhackable in their daily choices so they can *Reach Their Goals, Live Their Dream and Enjoy an Extraordinary Life*.

Your Next Steps with
Peripheral Neuropathy UNMASKED

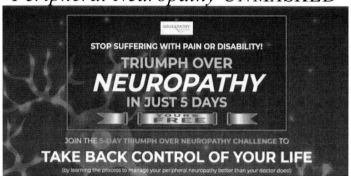

This Challenge is for you IF:

- If you want to... **UNDERSTAND** Your Peripheral Neuropathy Better Than Your Doctor Does
- If you want to... **MANAGE** The Symptoms of Peripheral Neuropathy Effectively
- If you want to... **CONTROL** The Nerve Damage So The Neuropathy Symptoms Stop Getting Worse
- If you want to... **LIVE** Your Dream Life Without The Distraction or Disability of Peripheral Neuropathy

When you are DIAGNOSED WITH PERIPHERAL NEUROPATHY often you are given few if any options for managing the symptoms, let alone improving the nerve function. Through this challenge you will learn to improve the Nerve Health and Stop the Nerve Pain.

https://www.treatmentforneuropathy.com

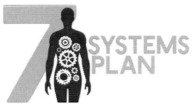

Are You Ready To Improve Your Health?

Utilizing the 7 Systems Plan, you can optimize all the systems of your body to improve your overall health and gain an unfair advantage over your Peripheral Neuropathy.

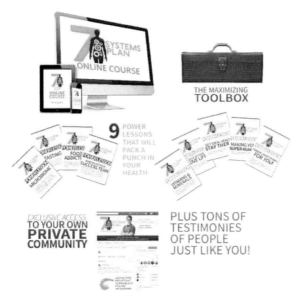

https://www.drbrandtgibson.com/7systems1

The Rebuilder™

Is it time to STOP the pain and numbness of Peripheral Neuropahty in your own home?

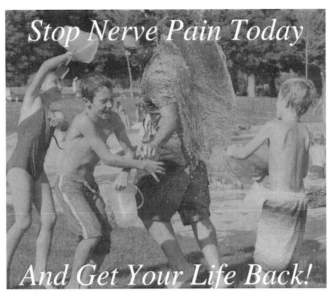

Get The Rebuilder™ Today
(for a special discount)

Get a FREE Foot Bath!

https://www.treatmentforneuropathy.com/rebuilder

USE THE SCIENCE OF PEAK PERFORMANCE
IN YOUR EVERYDAY LIFE

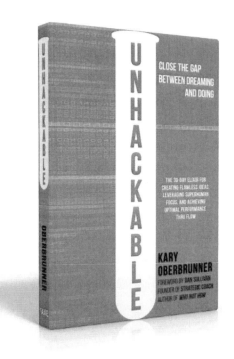

Get your <u>FREE Copy</u> of Kary Oberbrunner's Award Winning book and start BECOMING UNHACKABLE in all aspects of your life.

https://www.beunhackable.com/books

OTHER BOOKS IN THE *HEALTH UNMASKED SERIES*

Coming October 2021

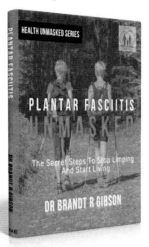

Coming October 2021

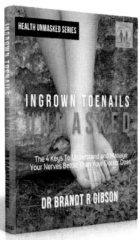

Coming November 2021

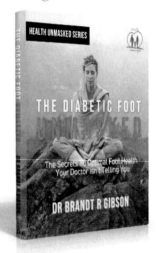

Coming December 2021

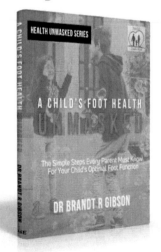

Coming December 2021

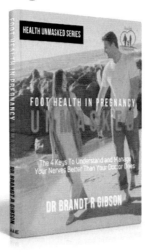

Made in United States
North Haven, CT
02 August 2022

22180971R00100